T0215345

LIBRARY COLLABORATIONS AND COMMUNITY PARTNERSHIPS

Library Collaborations and Community Partnerships illustrates the value of libraries and their resources through an array of alliances to improve health and enhance people's lives. It is unique in its illustration of key principles of collaboration, partner engagement, shared leadership, project development and outcomes measurement, as well as the challenges inherent in collaborations among diverse partners.

The book includes collaboration exemplars focused on education, health, information literacy and capacity building for populations that experience access and resource disparities. It highlights the innovative use of existing assets, environments and diverse professions to broaden access to resources and information to those in need. The strategies, challenges, outcomes and lessons learned that are described in the volume have application for a variety of settings and populations.

Highlighting the key role that libraries play in guiding successful interprofessional collaborations with communities, *Library Collaborations and Community Partnerships* should be of interest to academics, students and professionals engaged in library and information science, education, health care, social services and community organizations.

Vicki Hines-Martin is Professor and Assistant Dean, Office of Community Engagement and Diversity Inclusion at the University of Louisville, School of Nursing, Louisville, Kentucky, USA.

Fannie M. Cox is the Outreach and Reference Librarian, and Associate Professor, University of Louisville Libraries in Louisville, Kentucky, USA.

Henry R. Cunningham is the Director of Community Engagement at the University of Louisville, Louisville, Kentucky, USA.

LIBRARY COLLABORATIONS AND COMMUNITY PARTNERSHIPS

Enhancing Health and Quality of Life

Edited by
Vicki Hines-Martin, Fannie M. Cox
and Henry R. Cunningham

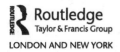
Routledge
Taylor & Francis Group

LONDON AND NEW YORK

First published 2020
by Routledge
2 Park Square, Milton Park, Abingdon, Oxon OX14 4RN

and by Routledge
52 Vanderbilt Avenue, New York, NY 10017

Routledge is an imprint of the Taylor & Francis Group, an informa business

British Library Cataloguing-in-Publication Data
A catalogue record for this book is available from the British Library

Library of Congress Cataloging-in-Publication Data
Names: Hines-Martin, Vicki, editor. | Cox, Fannie, editor. |
Cunningham, Henry R., editor.
Title: Library collaborations and community partnerships:
enhancing health and quality of life / edited by Vicki Hines-Martin,
Fannie Cox, and Henry R. Cunningham.
Identifiers: LCCN 2019058524 | ISBN 9781138343283 (hardback) |
ISBN 9781138343290 (paperback) | ISBN 9780429439261 (ebook)
Subjects: LCSH: Libraries and community. | Libraries and community—
United States. | Libraries and community—Case studies. |
Libraries and community—United States—Case studies. |
Libraries and society. | Libraries and education. | Library cooperation. |
Community leadership. | Interprofessional relations. | Public health.
Classification: LCC Z716.4 .L493 2020 | DDC 021.2—dc23
LC record available at https://lccn.loc.gov/2019058524

ISBN: 978-1-138-34328-3 (hbk)
ISBN: 978-1-138-34329-0 (pbk)
ISBN: 978-0-429-43926-1 (ebk)

Typeset in Bembo
by codeMantra

I would like to dedicate this book to my husband, Kenneth Martin, who loved me for 42 years, my daughter, Michelle, who continues to be my joy and my family with whom I could always find comfort and support. *Vicki-Hines Martin*

To my wife Unique Cox, thank you for your patience and support; to my parents James and Rosa, and my siblings who are no longer here – wish you were here to witness this accomplishment for which I dedicate to all of you.

And to my colleagues Drs. Vicki Hines-Martin and Henry R. Cunningham, thank you both for travelling this journey with me. Your work and commitment is monumental to making this book a reality. *Fannie M. Cox*

This book is dedicated to my wife Dr. Katie Matthews for her love and support, our darling and loving daughter, Marie, who brings great joy to our lives, and to my entire family for encouragement along the way. *Henry R. Cunningham*

CONTENTS

FIGURES

TABLES

CONTRIBUTORS

Ingrid Allard, MD, MSEd Ingrid Allard, MD, MSEd, is the Associate Dean for Community Outreach and Medical Education at Albany Medical College. She leads DivCOME and oversees the Service Learning Program.

Estanislado S. (Stan) Barrera IV, PhD, is an associate professor of literacy studies at Louisiana State University. His research is focused on bilingual literacy and improving teacher education. His research related to bilingual education concentrates on identifying and developing effective pedagogical approaches that maximize the students' "cultural capital" to achieve success. The roles of field experience and service-learning in developing pre-service teachers are the primary subjects of his research in regard to improving teacher education programs.

Maria Buhl, MLS, is the Department Head, Programs and Services/Interlibrary Loan at Guilderland Public Library. Over the last decade, Maria has collaborated with dozens of community organizations and providers to offer consumer health reference services to her patrons.

Kara Burke, MPH, is the Director for Community Engagement in DivCOME at Albany Medical College. She works closely with medical students and community partners to implement public health programs.

Hugh Burkhart (MA, University of Windsor; MLIS, University of Western Ontario) is an Associate Professor and the Coordinator of Instruction at the University of San Diego's Copley Library.

Mary K. Comtois is the Director of Health Initiatives at the United Way of Buffalo & Erie County. She is responsible for developing, managing, and leading strategic initiatives that produce improved health outcomes for residents of Buffalo and Erie County. Within this role, Mary K leads the Healthy Start Healthy Future for All Coalition and Human-Centered Design efforts within United Way.

Fannie M. Cox, MLS, MPA, is the Outreach and Reference Librarian, and Associate Professor, University of Louisville Libraries in Louisville Kentucky USA. In addition, Ms. Cox serves as the faculty liaison for the University's community engagement Signature Partnership Initiative and a liaison and Collection Development Specialist to the College of Education and Human Development, School of Urban and Public Affairs and Multicultural Children's collection at the University of Louisville. Ms. Cox earned her Bachelor of Arts (BA) and Master of Library Science from Indiana University, and a Master of Public Administration (MPA) from Kentucky State University.

Henry R. Cunningham, PhD, is the Director of Community Engagement at the University of Louisville, Louisville, Kentucky USA. He oversees all aspects of community engagement including policy, protocol, faculty development, and data collection and assessment. He also teaches a community-based learning course focusing on the Caribbean region. Dr. Cunningham has extensive background in international development and community engagement. He has conducted developmental work in several countries, and co-founded and co-directed the University of Louisville International Service Learning Program in addition to serving at the United Nations. He has published journal articles and book chapters on the topic of community engagement.

Montie' Dobbins, MLIS, is assistant director of technical services at the LSU Health Shreveport Health Sciences Library (LSUHS HSL). After obtaining her MLIS from Louisiana State University, she previously worked as Liaison Librarian and Head of User Access Services at LSUHS HSL.

David Duggar, MLIS, AHIP is the head of the library liaison program at the LSU Health Shreveport Health Sciences Library (LSUHS HSL). He earned his MLIS from Louisiana State University. Prior to his current position, he worked for LSU School of Veterinary Medicine Library as a General Librarian and LSU Health Sciences Center at Shreveport as a Reference Librarian. He has over 25 years of experience as a health sciences librarian.

Julia M. Esparza, MLS, AHIP, is the associate director of the LSU Health Shreveport Health Sciences Library (LSUHS HSL) and holds the Marianne & Stafford Comegys Professorship in Medical Library Science. After earning her MLS from Indiana University, she has worked in private, hospital, and academic libraries.

Enid Geyer, MLS, MBA, AHIP, is the Associate Dean for Information Resources and Technology and Director of SLHS at Albany Medical College. She is the principal investigator for this project.

Marilyn Harhai, MSLS, JD, PhD, is Professor in Department of Information and Library Science at Clarion University of Pennsylvania. Dr. Harhai is a faculty member in the MSLS program and teaches in the areas of collection development, literature, programming, and legal issues in libraries. She has worked in academic, public, and special libraries.

Julia Havey, RN, MSN, is Senior Systems Analyst at Loyola University Medical Center. Julia's experience related to the use of dogs in different settings is diverse. She has published on the quantifiable effects of animal-assisted therapy as it relates to pain medication use in post-operative patients. She has been a volunteer puppy raiser of service dogs for Canine Companions for Independence as a hands-on trainer and puppy raiser and educational demonstrator raising 23 dogs to date.

Gail Y. Hendler, MLS, is the director of the Loyola University of Chicago Health Sciences Library and has over 20 years of experience in public, hospital, and academic libraries. In addition to library administration, Gail teaches information mastery to students and faculty and frequently lectures on scholarly publication topics including copyright, Open Access, and predatory publishing. Gail obtained her master of library in information science from Queens College, City University of New York and has focused those skills on outreach, research, and education.

Vicki Hines-Martin, PhD, RN, FAAN, is Professor and Assistant Dean, Office of Community Engagement and Diversity Inclusion at the University of Louisville, School of Nursing, Louisville Kentucky, USA. Her work has focused on minority health, health disparities, community engagement and culturally sensitive intervention approaches in interprofessional programs and research initiatives. Dr. Hines-Martin is a Fellow in the American Academy of Nursing and Past-President of the International Society of Psychiatric Mental Health Nursing (2019–20). She has over 40 peer-reviewed articles and book chapters. Most recently she co-authored and edited – Yearwood, E., & Hines-Martin, V. P. Eds. (2016). *Routledge handbook of global mental health nursing: Evidence, practice and empowerment.* New York: Routledge/Taylor Francis Group.

Shane Hoffman is Technology Services Manager, Plain City Public Library. Shane loves his IT job where he gets to encourage SFSP participation, make musical instruments while watching Grizzly Adams and sometimes, fixing a computer.

Janet Ingraham-Dwyer is youth services library consultant at the State Library of Ohio. Her job is to provide support and resources for children and teen librarians and support staff in public and school libraries around the state. She manages Ohio's participation in the nationwide Collaborative Summer Library Program, fosters library participation in the Summer Food Service Program, and collaborates with the Ohio Library Council on Ohio Ready to Read, a statewide resource network to facilitate early literacy activities in libraries.

Elizabeth Irish, MLS, AHIP, is an Assistant Professor at SLHS, Albany Medical College. She has co-authored multiple publications and presentations on consumer topics.

Rita Kang, BSW, RSW, MEd, is Clinical Manager, Toronto Western Team Family Health Team – Garrison Creek (Formerly Corporate Manager, Patient Education and Engagement, University Health Network). Rita oversees clinical operations at a primary health clinic in Toronto, Ontario. She leads an interprofessional team, co-leads quality improvement initiatives, and develops community engagement strategies to improve access to primary care.

Caitlin Kelley was the Branch Supervisor of the Mason Square Branch Library from 2013 to 2019. She developed, planned, and orchestrated the branch's adult programming and many family-oriented programs and events, oftentimes in collaboration with community partners. Her programming efforts focused on community gardening, workforce development, access to legal services, art making for all ages, and concerts.

Elizabeth Kiscaden, MLIS, AHIP, NNLM GMR, is the Associate Director of the National Network of Libraries of Medicine (NNLM) Greater Midwest Region (GMR) office and has been a health sciences librarian for nearly a decade. Originally from Minnesota, Elizabeth worked at the Mayo Clinic in the Center for Translational Science Activities before relocating to Iowa.

Noah Lenstra, PhD, is an Assistant Professor of Library and Information Studies at the University of North Carolina at Greensboro School of Education. In 2016 he founded the project Let's Move in Libraries (http://letsmovelibraries.org/), focused on understanding how public libraries contribute to healthy physical activity through public programs. He received his PhD in Library and Information Science from the University of Illinois at Urbana-Champaign.

Jacqueline Leskovec, MLIS, MA, RN, NNLM GMR, has been with the National Network of Libraries of Medicine (NNLM) Greater Midwest Region (GMR) since 2005 and has served in various professional librarian capacities at both the previous Regional Medical Library (RML) at the University of Illinois at Chicago Library of the Health Sciences (Chicago, IL) and the current location at Hardin Library for the Health Sciences at the University of Iowa (Iowa City, IA).

Rosalind K. Lett, MBA, MLS, is the Director of the Clayton County Library System. She received her Bachelor of Sciences Degree in Life Sciences from Alabama A & M University, her Masters of Library and Information Studies from Atlanta University, and her Executive Master of Business Administration with emphasis on Global Leadership and International Business from Georgia State University.

Elizabeth Lynch is the Head of Teen Services at the Addison Public Library. She received her Master's in Library and Information Science from Dominican University in 2011, and has been working in public libraries since 2010. Elizabeth's work includes connecting teens to sexual and mental health resources, developing programming around social-emotional development, and adapting Restorative Justice models for the library setting.

Kelly MacGregor is the Community Engagement Department Head at the Berwyn Public Library. She received her master's degree in Library and Information Science from Dominican University in 2011, and has been working in public libraries since 2008. In that time, Kelly MacGregor has led several innovative initiatives, including becoming the first librarian in the state of Illinois to receive Department of Justice Accreditation, and designing Spanish language learning and enrichment activities for children and young adults from Spanish-speaking homes.

Phyllis Mancini, MA, Phyllis Mancini, MA, is a Health Communications Specialist, Patient Education & Engagement, University Health Network. Phyllis Mancini joined the University Health Network in 2005. She has a Master's degree in English and a background in adult education and communications. Phyllis supports clinicians and educators with their patient education needs by providing plain language workshops, consultations, and editing and publishing support with their educational materials (print or multimedia).

Lauren Manning is the Assistant Director at the Center for Law and Justice. She works to further the CFLJs mission of equity by engaging in strategic planning, community engagement, and working directly with clients to help them access needed resources.

Rebecca McFarland, MA, is a Community Initiatives Coordinator at the DuPage County Health Department. McFarland's work has centered on improving adolescent health outcomes.

Linda Miller, MPA, was formerly the Outreach and Education Coordinator at Community Caregivers, where she lead volunteer recruitment, training, caregiver education programming, and community outreach efforts.

Ophelia T. Morey, MLS, CHW is an associate librarian in the University Libraries at the University at Buffalo in Buffalo, New York, where her primary responsibility is community outreach. She is the recipient of several National Network of Libraries of Medicine funding awards.

William Olmstadt, MSLS, MPH, AHIP, is executive director of the LSU Health Shreveport Health Sciences Library (LSUHS HSL). He earned his MSLS from the University of Kentucky and an MPH from the University of Texas Houston School of Public Health. He has been a health sciences librarian for 19 years.

Christy Panagakis, PhD, is the Director of Research and Public Policy at the United Way of Buffalo and Erie County. She is responsible for researching the greatest sources of need in the Buffalo and Erie County community. In addition, she leads the organization's legislative advocacy efforts. She received her PhD in Sociology from the University at Buffalo in 2015.

Valeria Raivich, MLS, is Manager at Patient Learning & Experience Centres at the University Health Network (Formerly Librarian at the Patient & Family Library, Toronto Western Hospital, University Health Network). Valeria oversees four Patient & Family Libraries across University Health Network. She was a Librarian at Toronto Western Hospital for 13 years, where she provided direct customer service to the patients and was actively involved in patient education projects and health literacy promotion.

Brandon Reilly is the branch manager of Carver Branch Library in East Baton Rouge Parish Library System. Before accepting the position at Carver, he earned a masters of library science degree at Louisiana State University. Brandon shares his interest in library science with his wife, Leila, who is also a branch manager of a library in the East Baton Rouge Parish Library System.

Moira Rogers is Assistant Director for Latin America, CFHI, a first-generation Latina professional, holding a PhD in Science and Technology Studies, Virginia Tech. Her extensive teaching experience includes courses on Human Rights, Migration/Immigration, and Disabilities in a Global Context. Moira is passionate about developing and nurturing partnerships between the Global North and the Global South and about developing innovative strategies to expand access to international education for underrepresented students, faculty, and staff.

Nora Rose received a bachelor's degree in English from Barnard College of Columbia University prior to enrolling in the master's program in the School of Information at the University of Texas at Austin. She has held positions as writer, editor, group fitness instructor, and digital advertising strategist.

Loriene Roy, PhD, Professor in the School of Information, teaches in the areas of reference, library instruction/information literacy, and access and care of traditional knowledge. She served as the 2007–2008 President of the American Library Association.

Michael F. Russo received his MLIS from Louisiana State University in August of 2000. Since then and until 2016, he has worked for the LSU Libraries as a reference and instruction librarian. In 2016, he was made Collection Development and Analysis Librarian in the Collection Services department. He is a novelist and has written several peer-reviewed articles on various facets of library instruction.

Sarah Schaff is Discovery Librarian, Denison University. Sarah has had the good fortune to work in several Ohio Libraries since 2003, and now serves behind-the-scenes at a small, liberal arts college library, where weaving the threads of untold stories together has become one of her past-times. You can reach Sarah with thoughts about food insecurity, anti-hunger initiatives, and related notes at sarah@teamvittles.org.

Kim Skinner, PhD, is an associate professor of literacy and curriculum studies in the School of Education of Louisiana State University. Before teaching at the university level, she was a curriculum director, reading specialist, and classroom teacher of reading, writing, and language arts at the elementary level. Her research and teaching focus on how people use spoken and written language for learning in educational settings, and how people discursively construct knowledge, forge social relationships, and create communities.

Ellen Sulzycki is the Children's Services Supervisor for Springfield City Library and previously a Reference Librarian at Mason Square Branch Library. She loves to share ideas about learning and creating. She has been working with youth in libraries since 2013. Visit her online at ellenatthelibrary.com

Talicia Tarver, MLIS, AHIP, is currently a faculty librarian with Virginia Commonwealth University (VCU). With nearly ten years of health sciences library experience, Talicia graduated from Louisiana State University (LSU) in 2009 and worked for the LSU Health Shreveport Health Sciences Library (LSUHS HSL) for eight years before accepting a position as a Research and Education librarian for VCU. Talicia is currently the liaison for the VCU College of Health Professions.

Wilfrido Torres, MD, MPH, is Medical Director of CFHI Guayaquil & Puyo, Ecuador. He holds a degree in Medicine and General Surgery from the State University of Guayaquil and a master's degree in Clinical Investigation and Epidemiology. He is the Program Coordinator of the Vector Control Program with the Ministry of Public Health. He previously served as a primary care provider and ran a CFHI training program for health promoters in Indigenous villages outside of Puyo.

Cecilia Uribe de Chavez, MD, is Medical Director of CFHI La Paz, Bolivia. She is a Pediatrician with her own private practice, works at a municipal hospital in El Alto, and is the Secretary General of the Committee of Adolescents for the

Bolivian Society of Pediatrics. Dr. Uribe is the inspiration behind the Center for Empowerment of Young Mothers and is an expert on socio-economic determinants of health and healthcare delivery strategies in low-resource settings.

JoLynn Wheatley is the District Social Worker for Jonathan Alder Local Schools. She is a Licensed Independent Social Worker-Supervisor and Graduated with her master's degree in Social Work from The Ohio State University. She also obtained her School Social Work Certification.

Miu Lin Wong, MEd, RSSW, is an experienced health education specialist semi-retiring in Niagara Falls, Ontario. Before her retirement, she had worked in the Patient and Family Education Program, Toronto Western Hospital, University Health Network as Health Promotion Coordinator. She had initiated and developed numerous successful health education and promotion projects through meaningful internal and external partnerships including Monthly Health Talk.

Robin Young, MBA, is Director of Programs & Operations, CFHI. Robin's professional background includes extensive work in international education, global health, and asset-based development. She is the co-author of the Cultural Detective Dominican Republic series, and a Fulbright Fellowship grant recipient. Robin is passionate about supporting thoughtful, ethical, and asset-based strategies to address health disparities and support underserved communities.

Yan Zhang, PhD, is an Associate Professor in the School of Information at the University of Texas at Austin. She teaches in the areas of consumer health information, information architecture, software usability, and human factors in information retrieval.

ACKNOWLEDGMENTS

The following individuals reviewed the proposal for this book or various chapters of the book. We thank you for your expert thoughts and suggestions.

Prof. Ina Fourie
Department of Information Science
University of Pretoria
South Africa

Barbara A. Holland
Senior Scholar
Indiana University-Purdue University Indianapolis
United States

V. Faye Jones, MD, PhD, MSPH
Associate Vice President for Health Affairs/Diversity Initiatives
Professor of Pediatrics
Department of Pediatrics
University of Louisville
United States

Jim Neal
University Librarian Emeritus
Columbia University
United States

Joyce Neujahr
Director of Patron Services
University of Nebraska at Omaha

Dr. C.C. and Mabel L. Criss Library
United States of America

Dr. Lorraine J. Haricombe
Vice Provost and Director, University of Texas Libraries
University of Texas at Austin
United States

PART I
Theoretical foundations

1

INTRODUCTION

Vicki Hines-Martin

When many people think of libraries, they automatically think of quiet spaces, books, technology, and helpful people. Community members come to get help with research, education, or leisure pursuits. Sometimes they come to hear lectures or literary readings, or view films, and on special occasions there are book sales or activities for children. Libraries enrich our lives through these services. Although correct in many ways, this view is a very circumscribed one. The role of libraries is an advancing one within a changing paradigm.

Human development

The world is evolving in its perspective on how human development and human outcomes can be enhanced. Along with those changes has come the appreciation of the roles that libraries can play in this evolution. As organizations representing all disciplines and professions have identified, factors that influence individual, group, and community development and wellbeing are multifaceted and have a direct impact on the ability to enhance and transform our world. The United Nations has identified its agenda entitled *Transforming Our World: the 2030 Agenda for Sustainable Development* and identifies their goals as follows.

> To "seek to realize the human rights of all... (to address) three integrated and indivisible dimensions of sustainable development: the economic, social and environmental....to end poverty and hunger, in all their forms and dimensions, to ensure that all human beings can fulfil their potential in dignity and equality and in a healthy environment....to ensure that all human beings can enjoy prosperous and fulfilling lives and that economic, social and technological progress occurs in harmony with nature..... to mobilize the means required to implement this Agenda through a revitalised Global

Partnership for Sustainable Development, based on a spirit of strengthened global solidarity, focused in particular on the needs of the poorest and most vulnerable and with the participation of all countries, all stakeholders and all people. If we realize our ambitions across the full extent of the Agenda, the lives of all will be profoundly improved and our world will be transformed for the better.

(United Nations, 2015, pp. 3–4)

Key elements of *Transforming Our World: the 2030 Agenda for Sustainable Development* include a focus on achieving food security, ensuring healthy lives, and promoting wellbeing, fostering lifelong learning, and supporting human resilience, equality, social justice, and empowerment. Also significant to this document is the perspective that none of these goals can be accomplished by one group, entity, organization, or country. Critical to the agenda is implementing effective and targeted capacity building, evidence-based strategies which include "cooperation on and access to science, technology, innovation and enhance(d) knowledge sharing... through improved coordination among existing mechanisms" (United Nations, 2015, p. 31).

The World Health Organization (WHO) joined in the United Nations' effort by assuming a leadership role for *goal 3 to assure healthy lives and promote wellbeing for all ages.* The WHO identified that without health, the Sustainable Development Goals (SDGs) cannot be achieved and all the SDGs must be achieved in order to improve living conditions and, ultimately, human health and wellbeing. Human health and wellbeing is not only dependent on health services but also on all of the social, economic, and environmental determinants that influence opportunities, decision making, and outcomes among populations. Investment in health reduces poverty and contributes to economic growth, stronger human capital, and labor productivity. The WHO developed and endorsed their own 2030 Agenda companion document *Roadmap to implement the 2030 Agenda for Sustainable Development, building on Health 2020, the European policy for health and wellbeing* (2017) which included the following strategic directions, and enabling measures.

This roadmap proposes five interdependent strategic directions:

- Advancing governance and leadership for health and wellbeing
- Leaving no one behind
- Preventing disease and addressing health determinants by promoting multi- and intersectoral policies throughout the life-course
- Establishing healthy places, settings, and resilient communities
- Strengthening health systems for universal health coverage

It proposes four enabling measures to advance the implementation of both the 2030 Agenda and Health 2020:

- Investment for health
- Multi-partner cooperation

- Health literacy, research, and innovation
- Monitoring and evaluation

(WHO, 2017, p. 1)

Central to these foci is the use of existing networks and platforms to ensure dialogue between collaborating partners.

In the United States, former President Obama identified his commitment to the 2030 Agenda for Sustainable Development in a press release which identified that there was a need to leverage the full array of resources for development. It also sets forth the vision to use game-changing innovations and build sustainable systems to meet basic human needs (White House Office of the Press Secretary, 2015). President Obama identified that as a part of the international community

> there is a collective responsibility not only to help those in need, but to work together to address the root causes of poverty and conflict to ensure that all people have access to opportunity. ...it is incumbent upon all stakeholders – governments, the development community, faith-based organizations, research institutions, the private sector and ordinary citizens – to work together in partnership to contribute to a sustained global effort over the next 15 years, in order to deliver on the promise of this Agenda for our citizens.
> *(White House Office of the Press Secretary, 2015, p. 1)*

The United Nations 2030 Agenda had been widely accepted in Europe, the United States, and many other nations. How those goals would be enacted and accomplished was now a task which would be undertaken by many entities and organizations to support health and wellbeing among a variety of global populations and communities.

Human development and libraries

Those entities that have been consistently and prominently involved in supporting the health and wellbeing of their communities include **Libraries**. Libraries across the globe are a significant resource. The International Federation of Library Associations and Institutions identifies that there are approximately 2.5 million libraries worldwide, with most being school, public, academic, and community libraries (International Federation of Library Associations and Institutions, IFLA, n.d. [a]). On an international level the "International Federation of Library Associations and Institutions (IFLA) is the leading international body representing the interests of library and information services and their users. It is the global voice of the library and information profession" (IFLA, 2019). Their global vision is "a strong and united library field powering literate, informed and participative societies" (IFLA, n.d. [b]).

The IFLA has also committed to the United Nations 2030 Agenda and has published *Access and Opportunity for All – How Libraries Contribute to the United*

Nations 2030 Agenda (IFLA, 2016) outlining what they identify as their role in this global effort. They are committed to ensuring public access to information to protect fundamental freedoms, provide access and opportunity for all, and support universal literacy. These principles are enacted by libraries around the world using strategies which include services to support employment, public access to health information, safe environments for education focused on women's rights and entrepreneurial skills, and technology development. The focus of IFLA is to highlight the strengths of libraries as valuable collaborators in this complex effort and to identify libraries as critical leaders on a global stage.

Prior to the United Nations 2030 Agenda, the American Library Association began the *Libraries Build Sustainable Communities* Project in 2000 using the following perspective:

> The basic definition of "sustainable" is the use and stewardship of resources today that preserves them for tomorrow, and a sustainable community is one that is healthy and prosperous over the long term. The project defined three components of a sustainable community—Economy, Ecology, and Equity. Economy is the management, or stewardship, of the resources; Ecology is the relationship of the community with its environment, particularly the natural environment; and Equity is fairness to all.
>
> *(American Library Association, n.d. [a])*

Currently, The American Library Association supports and advances the IFLA Key Initiative 4.1 based on the United Nations 2030 Agenda (American Library Association, n.d. [a]).

4.1 *Promoting libraries within the United Nations 2030 Agenda for Sustainable Development*
     (which includes the following activities).

   Activity 4.1.2 *Change the mind set to achieve the vision of libraries as critical community assets;*
   Activity 4.1.3 *Campaign for Libraries in the United Nations 2030 Agenda for Sustainable Development;*
   Activity 4.1.4 *Develop evidence to demonstrate how access to information (A2I) and libraries contribute to the achievement of the Sustainable Development Goals (SDGs) outlined in the United Nations 2030 Development Agenda*
     (IFLA, n.d. [c])

The American Library Association (ALA) provides examples of the contributions of libraries in these broad areas (among others):

> Strengthening communities and facilitating community action through engagement

Meeting health and wellness needs through information and partnerships
Personal development through increased fiscal and computer literacy
Education within communities and academic settings

(American Library Association, n.d. [b])

ALA asserts that libraries are more than just storage spaces for books; libraries are important community hubs that serve as centers of learning and development, healthcare, and community building and support. The position that libraries hold as community anchors places library professionals in a unique position to be innovative in their approaches to serving the community. Both the IFLA and the ALA have clearly demonstrated the relevance of libraries to communities and how the work of libraries make them uniquely suited as partners and leaders in efforts for improvement of human development worldwide.

Because librarians are situated in, and part of, the communities they serve, they experience their communities firsthand, and can be the first to recognize an ongoing local need, issue, or priority as they interact on a daily basis with diverse visitors. Increasingly websites, blogs, and journal articles for public and professional education have identified and applauded the work of libraries and their staff as they assume this broader role to serve their communities and the areas in which libraries have expanded their reach are varied. For the homeless or the impoverished, libraries provide them with access to the technology and instruction through essential programs designed to help them move from poverty to self-sufficiency. Libraries are increasing the sites for health and wellbeing initiatives. Through their community programs, and direct staff assistance, libraries provide important equal access opportunities to those seeking to improve their health. Libraries and library professionals contribute two particular strengths to promote health: accessibility and trustworthiness. Many libraries address the needs of children and youth through the provision of much-needed safe spaces, addressing issues that affect their growth, development, and life skills, and providing access to resources. Libraries also help citizens gain needed skills and support to become advocates for themselves and their communities.

In conjunction with that expansion of services and roles within libraries has come the necessity for increased partnership with other organizations and entities to meet the complex needs and priorities of those communities. Together with governmental entities, healthcare providers and medical professionals, educational organizations, social services, and other environmental resources, libraries enhance communities and increase their resilience ways that make a significant impact.

Although there have been website, blog, and journal articles describing the communities, projects, outcomes, and research related to library-based initiatives, *Library Collaboration and Community Partnership: Enhancing Health and Quality of Life* presents in one volume a variety of library-led projects that illustrate a range in relation to types of projects, populations served, partnerships, and outcomes. In addition, the processes by which these projects were enacted are described along with the challenges and lessons learned as a result of their efforts. Contributors to this book also provide recommendations or considerations based upon their experiences for the benefit of the reader.

It should be noted that this book includes projects which are situated primarily within North America, with the majority coming from the United States. As a result, individual circumstances in which these projects are situated may be significantly different from those experienced by the reader. However, all presented material within this book falls within the frameworks which have been presented by the United Nations 2030 Agenda, the International Federation of Library Associations and Institutions (IFLA) Strategic Directions Key Initiative 4.1 as well as the American Library Association's Resolution on the Importance of Sustainable Libraries (American Library Association, 2015). Each of these documents has at their core the following important concepts:

1. Libraries in leadership as anchors within their communities
2. Library collaboration with others in innovative ways
3. Engaging with communities to identify needs, address issues, and improve outcomes

This book aims to discuss these principles that underlie the reported endeavors and provide a foundation for the reader as they examine the stories that are told. In addition we aim to demonstrate in some detail the processes by which each project was identified, undertaken, and evaluated through the lens of those principles. Through these presentations it is intended that the reader can identify an approach that will resonant and provide useful perspectives for consideration within the context of their resources or circumstance.

Library Collaboration and Community Partnership: Enhancing Health and Quality of Life is organized using the following format. Part I – Theoretical foundations – provides a discussion of the key elements of all of the presented library-led initiatives which includes libraries in leadership (Chapter 2), interprofessional collaboration (Chapter 3), and community engagement (Chapter 4).

Chapter 2 – Unrecognized roles of libraries in collaborations to improve communities – provides a historical and contextual discussion of the development of libraries and the expansion of the role of libraries within communities and settings. Chapter 3 – Interprofessional practice and collaboration – presents the evolving ideas around the definition and benefits of collaboration, and processes involved in collaborations across disciplines and professions. Chapter 4 – Communities and community engagement – describes critical elements of community partnership, the range of community engagement that can occur as projects are implemented, and the influence of community partnership on project outcomes and sustainability.

Part II includes library-led initiatives and research in the following categories: information literacy (Section A), education (Section B), health and behavior (Section C), and capacity building (Section D). Each of these sections begins with an introductory overview describing the overall focus of the exemplars that follow. The exemplars that are presented in each chapter provide examination of projects that may be viewed as familiar to the reader and those that are unique in their focus, approach, or population. In Part II, you will find that there is an overlap between chapters as it pertains to health-focused initiatives. Not only is health a significant need, how health needs are addressed varies. For example, some reported health projects focus on literacy, others on service provision partnership, still others on empowerment. Each demonstrates a different facet that was undertaken by the authors.

Part III – Perspectives, challenges, and future directions (Chapter 27) – provides a synthesis of the presented projects, identifies common challenges, and provides recommendations for future consideration.

The editors undertook the development of this book because of their interest in, and appreciation of, the contributions of libraries and librarians as collaborators and leaders in interprofessional projects for, and with, communities. The selected projects target a variety of audiences, from individuals who are novices to such collaborations to experts who wish to compare or validate their projects in relation to those that are reported here. Readers at any place on the spectrum should be able to benefit from the considerations and recommendations herein. Of particular value to any reader are the discussions and challenges of evaluation of the impact on the population served and the lessons learned. Description of these areas can function as guideposts for those interested in undertaking similar projects or enhancing current initiatives.

Lastly, this book is evidence of the value and strength of libraries and librarians in addressing the needs of communities for those professionals, organizations, and entities who have not had the benefit of their collaboration or who are unaware of their impact on health and wellbeing as well as sustainable communities.

References

American Library Association. (2015). Resolution on the importance of sustainable libraries 2014–2015 ALA CD#36_62815_FINAL. 2015 ALA Annual Conference. Retrieved from http://www.ala.org/aboutala/sites/ala.org.aboutala/files/content/governance/council/council_documents/2015_annual_council_documents/cd_36_substainable_libraries_resol_final.pdf

American Library Association. (n.d. [a]) Sustainability and libraries: Home. Retrieved from https://libguides.ala.org/SustainableLibraries

American Library Association. (n.d. [b]). Libraries matter. Retrieved from http://www.ala.org/tools/research/librariesmatter/category/building-strong-and-vibrant-community and http://www.ala.org/tools/research/librariesmatter/category/connecting-people-and-ideas

International Federation of Library Associations and Institutions-IFLA. (2016). Access and opportunity for all - How libraries contribute to the United Nations 2030 Agenda. Retrieved from https://www.ifla.org/files/assets/hq/topics/libraries-development/documents/access-and-opportunity-for-all.pdf

International Federation of Library Associations and Institutions-IFLA. (2019). About IFLA. Retrieved from https://www.ifla.org/about

International Federation of Library Associations and Institutions-IFLA. (n.d. [a]). Library map of the world. Retrieved from https://librarymap.ifla.org/map

International Federation of Library Associations and Institutions-IFLA. (n.d. [b]). Our vision, our future. Retrieved from https://www.ifla.org/node/11905

International Federation of Library Associations and Institutions-IFLA. (n.d. [c]). UN 2030 Agenda for sustainability development key initiative 4.1. Retrieved from https://www.ifla.org/node/10091

United Nations. (2015). Transforming our world: the 2030 Agenda for sustainable development A/RES/70/1. Retrieved from https://sustainabledevelopment.un.org/content/documents/21252030%20Agenda%20for%20Sustainable%20Development%20web.pdf

The White House Office of the Press Secretary. (2015). President Obama's commitment to global development - FACT SHEET: U.S. Global development policy and Agenda 2030. Retrieved from https://obamawhitehouse.archives.gov/the-press-office/2015/09/27/fact-sheet-us-global-development-policy-and-agenda-2030

World Health Organization Regional Committee for Europe. (2017). Roadmap to implement the 2030 Agenda for sustainable development, building on health 2020, the European policy for health and well-being EURO/RC67/9. Budapest, Hungary: WHO Regional Office for Europe. Retrieved from http://www.euro.who.int/__data/assets/pdf_file/0008/345599/67wd09e_SDGroadmap_170638.pdf

2

UNRECOGNIZED ROLES OF LIBRARIES IN COLLABORATIONS TO IMPROVE COMMUNITIES

Fannie M. Cox

Introduction

Is it safe to say that librarians like to share? This author thinks it must be second nature for librarians to share. At the Annual Conference of the American Library Association (ALA), there is a PR Xchange Event, along with the PR Xchange Awards Competition all focused on communication. Then, if you are on any one of ALA's CONNECT community listservs, of which there are over 300, it is rare that a week will go by without someone asking a question and a variety of responses pop-up, to share knowledge and/or experiences. Going back to library graduate school, all librarians are taught what it means to create new knowledge and how it allows librarians to add or share new knowledge to the profession, especially when there is a gap in the literature. Even with all these avenues for sharing, innovative programming, creative problem solving, new ideas, tools, and processes do not always get beyond the doors of the library. Because this is so, the exemplars in this book are being shared to highlight library's innovative use of existing assets through community partnerships and collaborations between diverse professions to broaden access to resources, programs, and information for those in need in a variety of settings and circumstances.

While there are books that discuss community engagement and outreach, this book will not only discuss those aspects, but it will describe strategies, challenges, outcomes, and lessons-learned with application for low-, middle-, and high-resource settings for a variety of populations. It will also serve as a resource that identifies how librarians and others have collaborated to make a difference to affect community health and quality of life. The work of libraries has evolved over time and has a rich history of responding to their user's needs in ways that enhance the lives of those who use them.

Library's history

Although libraries have existed for centuries, ancient libraries such as the Library of Ashurbanipal with its clay tablets during the 7th century BC in Iraq, the Libraries of Trajan's Forum around 112 AD in Rome, the House of Wisdom in the 9th century AD in Baghdad among others with their scrolls, each existed to serve their learned scholars and were not focused on use by the public.

The term public library had been used widely from the 17th century to refer to libraries open to the public that had been endowed by each of their benefactors. The first public library in the United Kingdom that was freely accessible to the public has been identified as one set up in the Free Grammar School in Coventry in 1601. The first library for public use in the United States is a topic of some discussion in the history books. Some have identified it as the Sturgis Library in Cape Cod in 1644. All libraries as we know them were enhanced by Johannes Gutenberg and his development of movable type which took the production of books into a new era. This new era in the United States was most commonly identified with Benjamin Franklin.

In 1731, the United States was a very young country with forward thinking leadership and very few resources including books, which were still being imported and were very expensive. Benjamin Franklin and several of his contemporaries joined together to establish the first subscription library, The Library Company of Philadelphia. Each member made monthly contributions to bring books to the colonies on a variety of subjects: politics, economics, social sciences, philosophy, religion, and the sciences to have intellectual discussions, address issues, and solve societal problems of that time (Wolf, 1976, p. 1). Thus began America's first formal library.

Since that time, the value of books and libraries has been well established in this country and their role in supporting all aspects of community and academic life is well documented. The first medical library, a special library, opened its doors in 1762 in the Pennsylvanian Hospital Library at the University of Pennsylvania. It is known as the Historic Medical Library. In 1847, it received the designation as the "first, largest, and most important medical library in the United States" by the American Medical Association (Historic Library, 1751). It preceded the United States Library of Congress (LC), which was founded in 1800. The oldest law library in the United States is the Jenkins Law Library, formerly known as the Law Library Company of the City of Philadelphia. It was founded in 1802 by its membership and continues to serve the legal community. Then in 1876, at the first American Library Association (ALA)[1] conference Samuel S. Green shared his idea of what makes the library a "useful institution". He stated that "personal relations between librarian and readers are useful in all libraries." Green described four functions that represent the core of what has become known as Public/Reference/User Services. Tyckoson's (2003) describes Green's four functions as:

- Instructing the reader in the ways of the library;
- Assisting the reader with his queries;

- Aiding the reader in the selections of good works; and
- Promoting the library within the community.

Within the four types of libraries: college and university, public, special, and school kindergarten thru 12th grade, only reference services are essentially unchanged. However, many other duties of librarians have expanded and evolved due to changes in the following areas: culture, economics, and social changes; the Internet and technological advances; and social media which have created new and exciting opportunities for libraries and their primary communities.

Opportunities for libraries

Outreach and community engagement have become embedded within the mission statement of many libraries and institutions of higher education, to collaborate and develop partnerships with communities and organizations outside the library and external to the University. For higher education, the objective is also to enhance the town-gown relationship between faculty and public communities through teaching, research, and service. Far too long, libraries have been an untapped resource. But the tide has begun to turn, because now many libraries are going beyond the traditional lending of books, videos, CDs, braille talking books, providing computers to apply for a job, and genealogy assistance to collaborating and forming partnerships to expand their reach locally, regionally, nationally, and internationally. In an information-rich environment, librarians are reinventing themselves to keep pace with users' needs and to justify their existence, especially when many libraries are experiencing budget shortfalls. Librarians are using data to drive decision-making, assessing their impact; demonstrate accountability, to justify why they are an asset to the communities they serve including academia. According to Bell's, "Staying True to the Core: Designing the Future Academic Library Experience" (Bell, 2014, p. 370),

> As technology advances, academic librarians must keep the [user] experience focused on the human elements of their relationship with community members while adapting it to a digital world of connected learning, artificial intelligence, and an Internet of Things, a future where every day physical objects will be connected to the Internet and able to exchange information with other objects.
>
> *(Bell, p. 370)*

The library has become much more user-centric and service oriented. These types of changes require librarians to meet their users where they are. While this is nothing new, it too requires librarians to continuously think about how they can meet the information needs and expectations of the communities they serve, and those communities that are in their service area, but have limited resources and broadband, yet need access to information. With this changing landscape, librarians continue to make the library "useful" (Green, 1876). The Library as place serves as both an anchor in the academic and the public community. So, how does the library transform itself to continue to support the information needs of its community and measure its impact on the community it serves?

Library communities, partnerships, and collaborations

The library is the "only centralized location where new and emerging information technologies can be combined with traditional knowledge resources in a user focused resource rich environment that supports today's social and educational patterns of learning, teaching and research" (Freeman, 2005). For academic libraries the term "community" has broadened to include not only students, faculty, and staff, who are the internal members of the academic community of the institution, but also the neighboring communities that surround the physical space of the library setting. Using Information Literacy as an outreach tool, libraries can transcend their university community to collaborate to exchange knowledge and resources through mutually beneficial and reciprocal partnerships to produce "engaged scholarship," "engaged teaching," or "engaged research," as an approach to align itself with the University's Community Engagement mission (Boyer, 1990). Information Literacy is defined as the "set of integrated abilities encompassing the reflective discovery of information, the understanding of how information is produced and valued, and the use of information in creating new knowledge and participating ethically in communities of learning" (American Library Association, 2015a).

Public libraries

In 2012b, ALA received a grant from the Institute of Museum and Library Services (IMLS) to advance library-led community engagement, "The Promise of Libraries Transforming Communities" (Bullard, 2012). Then in 2013b, ALA collaborated with the Harwood Institute, a leader in civic engagement to build a national plan and aligned it with the ALA's 2015 strategic plan, known as Transforming Libraries. The Urban Libraries Council (ULC) (2017, p. 2) analyzed survey data that identified an intersection between the last Great Recession which started around 2008 and the libraries becoming a "hub for economic opportunity." In addition, the ULC identified collaboration as one important strength of libraries: "Libraries are adept at building partnerships to support education goals. Partnerships include schools, workforce centers, colleges, federal agencies, high tech companies, civic organizations and nonprofits. Never the 'Lone Ranger', libraries seek out and thrive on partnerships that broaden impact" (Urban Libraries Council, 2015, p. 3). The library has become a place where one can also check out an outfit for an audition, graduation, prom, job interview, or some other formal event at the Grow Up Work Fashion Library of the New York Public Library (NYPL) Riverside Branch. At the NYPL Branch, library patrons can also checkout briefcases, neckties, and bowties from the, "Work Accessories Collection" and because of the library's social networking, patrons have access to professional stylist for assistance with clothing. In Pennsylvania, the University of Pennsylvania (Penn) reached out to the Free Library of Philadelphia to develop the partnership, the *Healthy Library Initiative*. The goal of the initiative was to "integrate evidence-based health efforts" (Morgan et al., 2016, p. 2030) using the library's existing structure of 54 branch libraries to promote and implement ten health programs in South Philadelphia's Community Health and Literacy Center. Penn recognized that working with public libraries provided an opportunity to promote and improve population health through the broad and diverse reach of Library patrons that frequent the libraries' many branches. Their collaboration produced an "engaged scholarship" product, a research article, *Beyond Books: Public Libraries as Partners for Population Health* (Morgan et al., 2016). Penn's study evaluated the ten programs implemented during the partnership. During the study period, there were "5.8 million in-person visits and 9.9 million online visits" recorded (Morgan et al., 2016, p. 2030), with 500,000 of those visits for specialized programming (Morgan et al., 2016, p. 2031). Patrons from different socioeconomic backgrounds, ages, educational level, immigrants, children and families, the homeless, those seeking information on mental health and substance use visited this library. More and more libraries are being called upon to form partnerships to assist in addressing societal issues of social justice, health, homelessness, and immigration. The next example of a partnership was a win-win situation both academically and for the public library. It provided an opportunity for students working towards the Masters of Social Work (M.S.W.) degree to set up shop at the library to hone their skills by fulfilling 900 hours of required fieldwork. According to Johnson (2019), the library is already known as a trusted and safe place in the community and the reported partnership allowed anyone to seek the services that MSW students could provide. For the library, it advanced its efforts to promote social justice, diversity, inclusion, and equity, while expanding its social service programming.

Universities and academic libraries

Libraries focused on higher education have also been on the cutting edge of innovation and experienced significant success through their partnerships in the areas of arts and humanities, business, the sciences, technology, health, and law. After all, Librarians as scholars "are the original collaborators in higher education" (Wilson, 2000). The literature clearly demonstrates that libraries are faced with a number of challenges affecting decisions related to budget, the design, delivery, and assessment of programs, and how best to use limited resources to address priorities focused on multiple stakeholders and consumers. In *Stormy Seas: The State of Library Budgets*, Scardilli (2015, p. 25) writes, "...libraries of all types have struggled in recent years to operate on limited budgets and redefine their roles as the world goes digital. The Great Recession that started in 2008 put many libraries on a downward slope." The demands of accreditation and standards have forced academic institutions to recognize Information Literacy (IL) more fully within the context of the broader educative community as vital to student learning. While students' and academic changing needs and expectations compound the difficulty, librarians have sought to develop more dynamic and diverse approaches in collaboration with other disciplines (Brasley, 2008; Miller et al., 2010; Travis, 2008).

How library collaborations can contribute to communities

Collaboration is an important learned behavior. Librarians have long understood the importance of relationship building due to their long history of providing programming, working with communities they serve and support, and building cooperative relationships amongst each other. Diverse talents and a wide array of resources are brought together to solve a problem, build a program, or create something entirely new (Boyer, 1990). The goal is to build and bridge relationships to form social networks that not only strengthens our society, but enhances quality of life and improve communities. In many library collaborations, the transdisciplinary approach often occurs organically to solving social civic, economic, and moral problems when more than two types of knowledge/disciplines converge to create new knowledge and/or solutions. Collaboration is discussed further in Chapter 3.

Hang Tat Leong's article, *Community Engagement – Building Bridges between University and Community by Academic Libraries in the 21st Century* (2013), examined 18 large academic libraries in the United States, Canada, and China and found that academic libraries primarily focused on four types of outreach: (1) community access; (2) information literacy; (3) cooperation, exchange, and partnership; and (4) exhibitions and scholarly events. The author also reviewed each university's mission statement for evidence of outreach or community engagement and found that community engagement and outreach is emphasized by universities around the world. Serials management provided an opportunity for an international institutional exchange partnership between Appalachian State University (ASU) in Boone, North Carolina, USA and libraries in China. They participated in discussions, found their common interests, and worked out a plan to assist the other on serials staffing, collection development, and budgeting (Leong, 2013, p. 227). Similar exchange programs have occurred between the American University in Afghanistan (AUAF) and universities in Qatar's Education City, where the librarians met with their counterparts and shared experiences. Academic libraries build bridges, by using the library's resources, its collections, space, service-oriented staff, and technology, to build partnerships with scholars and the public community as a means of fulfilling the university's emphasis on community engagement and outreach.

Louisville, Kentucky USA is home to the Wayside Christian Mission's (WCM) Hotel Louisville facility. This facility is a working hotel that receives guests from all over the country. It is also a homeless transition shelter for families working to become self-sufficient. Within Hotel Louisville, two floors have been set aside to house homeless women and their children as residents of this program. These families who reside and work within the hotel learn hospitality employment skills and are provided wrap-around family services to support their ability to be self-sustaining and independent members of the community. With its multiple programs and facilities, WCM utilizes a holistic approach to get to the fundamental causes of homelessness experienced by men, women, and children of metropolitan Louisville, Kentucky. Several unique projects occur simultaneously within this setting. One library-led collaboration focuses on increasing resident literacy – *Using Technology and Information Literacy to Engage the Homeless* (Cox, 2013).

Wayside residents were participants in Wayside's College and Career Program and were preparing to begin an orientation to technical college class. As preparation, Wayside 100 was developed and implemented as a basic computing and information literacy skills class to help the students reach the needed college-level skills. The class included internet basics, keyboarding, beginning word processing, opening an email account, creating or updating a resume, and applying for employment online. The library – Wayside collaborative was both unique and innovative.

Library challenges: new jobs, new duties, new realities, and community engagement

Historically, anyone who needed something from the library had to go into the physical setting for assistance to access many of the libraries resources and collections. Today, access to many of the library's resources is available digitally, conveniently in the privacy of one's home, office, or mobile device. Vast amounts of information are available on the Internet. Now more than ever, especially in an era of "fake news," information literacy (IL) should be mandatory throughout the educational process. As change occurs, libraries regardless of setting are reviewing their roles and reflecting on their contributions to determine their importance, relevance, efforts, and outcomes with less funding, staff, space, etc., while competing with other entities (i.e. public/private businesses, non-profits, politics, the market place, etc.) for respect, acknowledgment, and financial support. New roles that were once uncommon in Librarianship have now become commonplace.

The library landscape has changed in all manner of ways – job titles and expectations, responsibilities, access, and delivery of services, to name a few. However, the Digital Divide is alive and well with, many people facing additional barriers to educate and equip themselves with life's basic necessities. For the librarian, it can mean updating one's skill set(s) to stay current with the ever-changing backdrop of the community they serve. Many libraries have development positions for fund-raising; public relations positions to create a "brand" for marketing purposes; research data management (RDM) and data curator positions to assist the professions such as STEAM (science, technology, engineering, arts, math), medical professionals, and academicians with their data management plans, digital repositories, and open access (OA) publishing.

The library is where many things are possible. When challenges arise, the place to turn can be the library. In 2015, Baltimore, Maryland's Pennsylvania Avenue Branch of the Enoch Pratt Free Library was ground zero when a massive protest broke out against police brutality. A CVS drugstore across the street from this library was looted and torched. Nevertheless, the Branch remained opened and served its community. The library was untouched by the hostility (American Libraries, 2015). Community members recognized the library as a safe haven – the place where one can go for assistance to find traditional services, such as learning how to read, printing, to find information about a job, or use the computer; and non-traditional services where people can go during a community crisis, find health services, a social worker, clothing and accessories for an interview, or the prom.

Libraries contributions to the academy, community, and global impact

To conclude, society has not realized the full potential of libraries. Libraries are an asset to any community. Through community engagement and outreach, opportunities exist for partnerships and collaborations with unimaginable and infinite possibilities. While crises and challenges are barriers for some, they can be opportunities for libraries to develop non-traditional programs, even with limited budgets, personnel, and space. Libraries persevere.

Note

1 As the largest and oldest professional membership-driven library association in the world, the America Library Association (ALA) was founded in 1876. The organization represents libraries according to type and/or function through its 11 divisions and networks of library community supporters, chapters, affiliates, schools P-16, academic, government, corporate and public organizations. It has more than 55,000 members.

References

ALA. (2012a). ALA Midwinter conversations: Community engagement and the promise of libraries transforming communities. Retrieved from http://www.ala.org/news/press-releases/2012/11/ala-midwinter-conversations-community-engagement-and-promise-libraries

ALA. (2012b, March 5) Empowering voices, transforming communities: An initiative of ALA President Molly Raphael. Retrieved from http://www.ala.org/advocacy/advleg/empoweringvoices

American Library Association (ALA). (2013a). ALA President Barbara Stripling unveils 'declaration for the right to libraries'. Retrieved from http://www.ala.org/news/

press-releases/2013/07/ala-president-barbara-stripling-unveils-declaration-right-libraries

ALA. (2013b). The promise of libraries transforming communities: A presidential initiative. Retrieved from http://www.americanlibrariesmagazine.org/inside-scoop/promis-libraries-transforming-communities-presidential-initiative

American Library Association. (2015a). About: ACRL releases new roles for the road ahead (https://www.jenkinslaw.org/about). Retrieved from http://www.ala.org/news/press-releases/2015/03/acrl-releases-new-roles-road-ahead

American Library Association (ALA). (2015b, February 9). Framework for information literacy for higher education. Retrieved from http://www.ala.org/acrl/standards/ilframework

Bell, S. (2014). Staying true to the core: Designing the future academic library experience. *Libraries and the Academy, 14*(3), 369–382.

Boyer, E. L. (1990). *Scholarship reconsidered: Priorities of the professoriate.* Princeton, NJ: Princeton University Press, The Carnegie Foundation for the Advancement of Teaching.

Brasley, S. S. (2008). Effective librarian and discipline faculty collaboration models for integrating information literacy into the fabric of an academic institution. *New Directions for Teaching and Learning, 2008*(114), 71–88. doi:10.1002/tl.318

Bullard, G. (2012, October 5). The promise of libraries transforming communities. Press Release, Washington, DC: The Institute of Museum and Library Services. Retrieved from https://www.imls.gov/news/imls-awards-ala-grant-advance-library-led-community-engagement

Cottrell, M. (2015, May 1). Baltimore's library stays open during unrest: Q&A with CEO Carla Hayden. *American Libraries.* Retrieved from https://americanlibrariesmagazine.org/blogs/the-scoop/qa-carla-hayden-baltimore/

Cox, F. M. (2013). Engaging the homeless through technology and information literacy. *Metropolitan Universities: An International Forum, 24*(3), 1–124.

Freeman, G. T. (2005). Libraries as place: Changes in patterns, collections, technology and use. In *Libraries as place: Rethinking roles, rethinking space* (pp. 1–10). Washington, DC: Council on Libraries and information resources.

Freeman, G. T., Bennett, S., Demas, S., Frischer, B., Peterson, C. A., Oliver, K. B., & Council on Library and Information Resources, W. D. (2005). Library as place: Rethinking Roles, rethinking space. Council on Library and Information Resources, Washington, D.C

Green, S. S. (1876, October 1). Personal relations between librarians and readers. *Library Journal,* (1993), *118*(11), pS5, 2. Retrieved from http://echo.louisville.edu/login?url=https://search.ebscohost.com/login.aspx?direct=true&db=llf&AN=502787199&site=ehost-live

Johnson, S. C. (2019). MSW interns and public libraries: Enhancing services through interdisciplinary collaboration. *Public Services Quarterly, 15*(1), 13–23. doi:10.1080/15228959.2018.1541332

Leong, J. H. T. (2013). Community engagement – Building bridges between university and community by academic libraries in the 21st Century. *Libri, 63*(3), 220–231. doi:10.1515/libri-2013-0017

Miller, L. C., Jones, B. B., Graves, R. S., & Sievert, M. C. (2010). Merging silos: Collaborating for information literacy. *Journal of Continuing Education in Nursing, 41*(6), 267–272. doi:10.3928/00220124-20100401-03

Morgan, A. U., Dupuis, R., D'Alonzo, B., Johnson, A., Graves, A., Brooks, K. L., ... Cannuscio, C. C. (2016). Beyond books: Public libraries as partners for population health.

Health Affairs (Project Hope), 35(11), 2030–2036. Retrieved from https://search.ebsco host.com/login.aspx?direct=true&db=cmedm&AN=27834243&site=ehost-live

Scardilli, B. (2015). Stormy seas: The state of library budgets. *Information Today, 32*(10), Cover-27. Retrieved from http://echo.louisville.edu/login?url=https://search.ebsco-host.com/login.aspx?direct=true&db=c8h&AN=111720016&site=ehost-live

Travis, T. (2008). Librarians as agents of change: Working with curriculum commit-tees using change agency theory. *New Directions for Teaching & Learning*, 114, 17–33. doi:10.1002/tl.314

Urban Libraries Council. (2015). Libraries and economic opportunity. White Paper. Re-trieved from https://www.urbanlibraries.org/files/ULC_White-Papers_LIBRARIES-AND-ECONOMIC-

Wilson, B. (2000). The lone ranger is dead. *College & Research Libraries News, 61*(8), 698. Retrieved from http://echo.louisville.edu/login?url=https://search.ebscohost.com/login.aspx?direct=true&db=lxh&AN=3735690&site=ehost-live

Wolf, E. (1976). *"At the instance of Benjamin Franklin": A brief history of the library company of Philadelphia 2nd Ed, 1731–1976.* Philadelphia, PA: Library Company of Philadelphia.

3

INTERPROFESSIONAL PRACTICE AND COLLABORATION

Vicki Hines-Martin

In this book, collaboration is a critical component of each of the projects that is presented. Individuals who have expertise in library science have routine experiences in which they partner with the public using their unique knowledge. That specialized knowledge has also become increasingly recognized as a valuable asset in research and educational development for those individuals and organizations in the sciences and professions. The exemplars in this text clearly illustrate the critical nature of library partnerships in projects which are both *routine* and *unique*, truly reflecting the meaning of the term "exemplar". A core concept in partnerships focused on development, implementation and successful outcomes in any endeavor is **collaboration**. Whether the partnerships are formal or informal, brief or ongoing in nature, the mechanisms by which each member of the partnership functions involves collaboration. The term collaboration is often used; however, its definition has varied over time and discipline.

The terms cooperation and collaboration are often times used interchangeably. However, there are some important differences between the two terms. Mattessich and Monsey (1992) define *cooperation* as joint relationships that exist without any commonly defined objective, organization or design; meanwhile *collaboration* changes previously separate entities into a new structure with dedicated efforts to a common outcome (Mattessich & Monsey, 1992). Schrage (1995) identifies that collaboration involves a process that results in two or more individuals or organizations with complementary skills interacting to create a shared understanding and goal that is uniquely different than what they had as a single entity to achieve a distinctive outcome (Podean et al., 2011; Schrage, 1995; Shelbourn et al., 2007). Thomson and Perry (2006) and Thomson et al. (2007) stress that collaboration develops over time, while participants interact formally and informally with each other to create new processes and systems.

Collaboration may occur at any level of an organizational structure. People can collaborate between two or more individuals, within or between organizations, communities as well as separate countries. *Within this text, collaboration is a shared association with a common vision to create a joint project based on key elements of trust and transparency, with the goal to enhance an identified outcome for a targeted population.* This is accomplished by addressing common concerns or goals using bidirectional communication and planning, and by sharing responsibilities, challenges and rewards. The literature from a variety of disciplines and professions identify that what results from this type of collaboration was improved outcomes to address complex problems within organizations and society. Because these challenges are multifaceted they cannot be fully addressed by a single discipline or profession but require expertise and perspectives from multiple disciplines and this need continues to grow as our world becomes increasingly complex. Along with increased complexity are environmental resource constraints such as money, personnel, technology and facilities. Collaboration can facilitate the more efficient and effective use of these limited resources. As partnerships form they require greater flexibility and innovation in order to be successful (Bart & Johnson, 2015; Keck et al., 2017). Schöttle et al. (2014) identified the following components for a successful collaboration (see Figure 3.1).

They also identify critical elements in collaborative membership which greatly influence the chances of successful collaboration. These are members who hold mutual respect for the skills of other partners, mutual understanding of the value and appropriateness of the partner's skills to achieve the desired outcomes, and the ability to trust that those desired are mutual. Although collaborations among various entities have commonality in purpose, they may be different in the extent to which they collaborate. These collaborations are identified by terms such as *interdisciplinary* as well as *interprofessional* collaborations in the literature. These

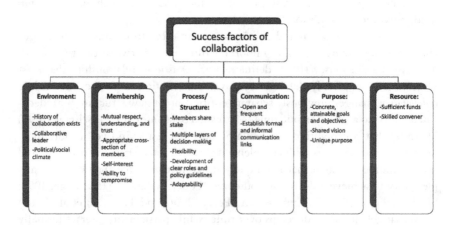

FIGURE 3.1 Success factors of collaboration.
Source: Schöttle, Haghsheno & Gehbauer (2014). Used with permission.

terms have both similarities and dissimilarities and some distinctive characteristics that have implications for their use and applicability.

The term **interdisciplinary** was first discussed in the literature in 1972 (Jantsch, 1972) and identified the need for social science in academic settings to function in a more collaborative way to answer scientific questions and teach through the integration of knowledge and methods among the various disciplines. Through this interdisciplinary approach, it was demonstrated that a more holistic perspective was accomplished resulting in innovation in outcomes. Since the development of the concept of interdisciplinary collaboration, there has been evolution in defining degrees of interdisciplinary collaboration resulting in three distinct classifications: **multidisciplinary, cross-disciplinary** and **transdisciplinary** collaborations.

Miller (2017) presents the following classifications for interdisciplinary collaborations based on the literature.

> **Multidisciplinary** approaches involve the simple act of juxtaposing parts of several conventional disciplines in an effort to get a broader understanding of some common theme or problem. The disciplines do not need to change any of their protocols, and yet they can claim their openness to interdisciplinary cooperation (p 8)… **Crossdisciplinary** approaches involve real interaction across conventional disciplines, though the extent of communication and thus combination, synthesis, or integration of concepts and/or methods varies considerably.....six sub-category of crossdisciplinary approaches are: (a) topics of social interest, (b) professional preparation, (c) shared analytical methods, (d) shared concepts, (e) hybrids and (f) shared life experiences (p 8).. **Transdisciplinary** approaches have been understood to involve articulated conceptual frameworks that seek to transcend the more limited worldviews of the specialized conventional disciplines. Advocates for transdisciplinary approaches often directly challenge the efficacy of conventional disciplines, claiming that they are part of the problem rather than the solution, especially when the objective is the mitigation of complex social problems.
>
> *(Miller, 2017, p. 11)*

As is reflected in the above definitions, the depth and breadth of the collaborations change according to category with the relationships becoming more involved and participants who are part of that interactive relationship involving not only those with specialty expertise but also those who are stakeholders in the desired outcomes including populations and communities.

Collaboration principles in the health professions are similar to those described above and are often referred to as **interprofessional collaboration** (IPC). Interprofessional collaboration also encompasses important key concepts such as partnership, interdependency and shared power. In health care, it is generally believed that collaborative efforts yield better health services and outcomes for the populations served. Littlechild and Smith (2013) state that collaboration leads to improved efficiency, improved skills mix, greater levels of responsiveness, more holistic services, innovation and creativity, and a more user-centered practices. The World Health Organization (WHO) has linked IPC with better outcomes in family health, infectious disease, humanitarian efforts, responses to epidemics and noncommunicable diseases (WHO, 2015). The research literature has demonstrated advances in access to care, and coordination of services, appropriate use of specialty care, chronic disease outcomes and safety (Lemieux & McGuire, 2006; WHO, 2015). Important indicators such as complications and error rates, length of hospital stay, conflict among caregivers, staff turnover and mortality rates have all exhibited decreases in collaborative care environments (WHO, 2015).

It has been suggested in the literature that IPC practice is different from interdisciplinary, multidisciplinary and transdisciplinary practice. Discussion of IPC has been applied to collaborations that provide care to populations or communities whereas interdisciplinary, multidisciplinary and transdisciplinary practice care provided by more than one health care provider for the benefit of a patient rather than an entire population or community (Boon et al., 2004; Johnson, 2009; Stone, 2009). IPC relies upon the integration of people not often associated with health care, who may assist in improving health care outcomes of a targeted group being served with an awareness of the social and environmental factors that impact health. In an IPC collaboration, the input of social services, informatics and library specialists, technology experts and others may be essential to a successful outcome. Some of the exemplars presented in this text illustrate this broader application of IPC.

Interorganizational collaboration is differentiated as a set of processes in which professionals representing multiple organizations engage in working interdependently on a designated intervention towards an outcome (Keyton et al., 2008). In health care, the promotion of interorganizational collaboration is becoming a top priority for policy makers and regulatory bodies in order to move towards coordinated structures to provide efficient, high-quality services in community settings. Interprofessional collaboration is an integral part of successful interorganization collaboration. However, interprofessional collaboration may occur in the absence of interorganization collaboration. Karam et al. (2018) in their synthesis of the literature identified the following shared and distinct characteristics of interprofessional and interorganizational collaboration. Shared characteristics include influence of the external environment on the development and implementation of collaboration, inherent essential factors (trust, power and mutual acquaintanceship), communication, tasks foci (shared goals and user-centeredness) and targeted outcomes. Distinct characteristics of interprofessional collaboration are internal environmental factors, and role flexibility among individuals within the team. Distinct characteristics of interorganizational collaboration are identified as process formalization and professional role clarification as preparation for ongoing functioning (Karam et al., 2018). Green and Johnson (2015) proposed a checklist to assess for an organization's readiness for collaboration (see Table 3.1).

Although this check list is viewed as an organization's self-assessment, it requires discussion and exploration of all organizational partners to adequately complete

TABLE 3.1 Checklist to assess for an organization's readiness for collaboration from Green and Johnson (2015). Used with permission

Readiness for Collaboration	*Yes*	*No*

1. Would the situation (research, education, outreach or clinical issue) of interest be best solved through collaboration?
2. Who should be included in the collaboration? Are the appropriate collaborators (disciplines, services and professions) being considered and invited?
3. Have you identified the benefits that each of the collaborators will gain from the relationship?
4. Have you identified the potential barriers to working effectively (e.g. culture, vocabulary, approaches, distance, technology, etc.)?
5. Have you developed a plan for how these barriers will be overcome?
6. Have the following been assessed for key team members regarding collaboration: attitudes, environmental concerns, communications, resources and trust?
7. Have you considered the intangible elements for each collaborator (e.g. tacit knowledge, social capital, transparency, motivation)?
8. Have the organizational outcomes been clearly stated and agreed upon (what do you hope to produce from the collaboration)?
9. Is there support and commitment across all levels for this collaboration to be successful, including administrators, collaborators and involved personnel?
10. Have all members of the collaborative team agreed upon the goals and the shared purpose?
11. Does everyone in the collaboration have adequate and available time, resources and skills in order to accomplish the goals?
12. Is there an overt environment and culture of mutual respect amongst all members? If not, what is the plan to develop this?
13. Have you developed and agreed upon the plan to manage and resolve conflict or disagreement when it occurs?
14. Have the collaborators agreed to share in all of the following: planning, decision making, problem solving, evaluation responsibility, working together cooperatively, communicating and coordinating openly?

the assessment. Through this assessment process, the collaborators also begin formulating their roles, identifying complementary skills and desired outcomes.

Collaborative approaches have become more common as part of graduate health professions education and benefits have been demonstrated in student scholarship. Research has identified that graduate students who were in transdisciplinary training groups published in higher impact journals were more frequently cited and had more cross-disciplinary collaborations (Keck et al., 2017). In the conduct of research, collaborating parties benefit not only in accomplishing research studies that further understanding of complex phenomenon but also in building networks, encouraging different thinking, stimulating and utilizing approaches that could not be accomplished by a single profession through the integration of a variety of professionals as part of the learning process.

Even as collaborations have been discussed in terms of purpose and benefits to collaboration participants and targeted populations, these collaborations also come with the need for identification of appropriate strategies by which outcomes can be measured at many levels and from different perspectives. Collaboration outcomes are amenable to investigation through traditional research methods or program evaluation. Because of the complexity of collaborations, measurement of outcomes frequently involves a combination of these two approaches or a single focus on evaluation. Research which is focused on the development of knowledge may target the end user or product resulting from the collaboration, whereas evaluation is used to assess the processes and outcomes of a specific initiative and must consider the contributions and perspectives of the diverse participants involved in the collaboration and may focus on the process, the outcome and the impact of the collaboration. This evaluation takes into consideration each phase of the collaborative effort – planning, implementation, completion, dissemination and information sharing and should include input from all stakeholders especially the recipients of those collaborations. Organizations that focus on research and evaluation of multi-partner collaborations involving professionals and communities identify the challenges and the need for assessment according to the agreed upon values and mutual priorities for the project (Clinical and Translational Science Award Consortium Community Engagement Key Function Committee Taskforce on the Principles of Community Engagement, 2011; Committee on Evaluating Quality Outreach, 2000; Thomson et al., 2007). The Committee on Evaluating Quality Outreach (2000) identifies critical dimensions for evaluation that are found in the literature on collaboration – significance or importance of the project, content of the project and impact on the targeted population based upon the established values and mutual priorities. As the literature about collaborations grows, a fourth dimension is key – that of scholarship (Committee on Evaluating Quality Outreach, 2000).

Although the discussion of collaborations has increased in the literature since 1990s, it has primarily been focused on the social sciences, business, technology and health. Collaboration regardless of its type is now part of the lexicon among research, professional practice/service and education when strategies are discussed to address the needs of groups, populations and communities. This increase has resulted in a corresponding rise in literature from other disciplines regarding the development, challenges and successes of collaborative projects. More recently, collaborations with libraries has joined this growing body of literature. The literature includes discussion of library collaborations as part of research teams, scholarship and creative work and writing (Brandenburg et al., 2017; García-Millian et al., 2013; Janke & Rush, 2014; Newell, 2007; Thomas & Leonard, 2014; Wilkes & Miodownik, 2018). However, libraries serve in a broader capacity in a variety of collaborations to address population and community needs, many of these collaborations are led by libraries themselves. *Library, collaboration and community partnership: Enhancing health and quality of Life* presents collaborations between libraries and their partners in the areas of literacy, health and empowerment to provide services, technology, education and support to a variety of communities and populations. These collaborations vary across the spectrum reflecting those that have been discussed in this chapter. The book's exemplars provide real-world demonstrations of how collaborations with libraries are developed and function towards desired outcomes. The presented projects discuss their challenges, approach to evaluation, lessons learned and recommendations that raise awareness of the daily contributions of libraries as collaborative partners. The exemplars will also discuss the innovations that can and do result from collaboration with libraries in a variety of settings that are both common place and unique.

References

Bart, B. N., & Johnson, C. D. (2015). Interprofessional collaboration in research, education, and clinical practice: working together for a better future. The Journal of chiropractic education, 29(1), 1–10. https://doi.org/10.7899/JCE-14-36

Boon, H., Verhoef, M., Ohara, D., & Findlay, B. (2004). From parallel practice to integrative health care: A conceptual framework. *BMC Health Services Research, 4*(1), doi:10.1186/1472-6963-4-15

Brandenburg, M., Cordell, S., Joque, J., MacEachern, M., & Song, J. (2017). Interdisciplinary collaboration: Librarian involvement in grant projects. *College & Research Libraries, 78*(3), 272. doi:10.5860/crl.78.3.272

Clinical and Translational Science Awards Consortium Community Engagement Key Function Committee Task Force. (2011). *Principles of community engagement -2nd edition*. Retrieved from https://www.atsdr.cdc.gov/communityengagement/pdf/PCE_Report_508_FINAL.pdf

Committee on Evaluating Quality Outreach. (2000). *Points of distinction: A guidebook for planning & evaluating quality outreach*. Lansing: Michigan State University.

García-Millian, R., Norton, H. F., Auten, B., Davis, V. I., Holmes, K. L., Johnson, M., & Tennant, M. R. (2013). Librarians as part of cross-disciplinary, multi-institutional team projects: Experiences from the VIVO collaboration. *Science and Technology Libraries, 32*(2), 160–175. doi:10.1080/0194262X.2013.791183

Green, B. N., & Johnson, C. (2015). Interprofessional collaboration in research, education, and clinical practice: Working together for a better future. *Journal of Chiropractic Education, 29*(1), 1–10. doi:10.7899/JCE-14-36

Janke, R., & Rush, K. (2014). The academic librarian as co-investigator on an interprofessional primary research team: A case study. *Health Information and Libraries Journal, 31*, 116–122. doi:10.1111/hir.12063

Jantsch, E. (1972). Towards interdisciplinarity and transdisciplinarity in education and innovation. In L. Apostel (Ed.), *Interdisciplinarity: Problems of teaching and research in universities* (pp. 97–120). Paris, France: CERI/OECD.

Johnson, C. (2009). Health care transitions: A Review of integrated, integrative, and integration concepts. *Journal of Manipulative and Physiological Therapeutics, 32*(9), 703–713. doi:10.1016/j.jmpt.2009.11.001

Karam, M., Brault, I., Durme, T. V., & Macq, J. (2018). Comparing interprofessional and interorganizational collaboration in healthcare: A systematic review of the qualitative research. *International Journal of Nursing Studies, 79*, 70–83. doi:10.1016/j.ijnurstu.2017.11.002

Keck, A. S., Sloane, S., Liechty, J. M., Fiese, B. H., & Donovan, S. M. (2017). Productivity, impact, and collaboration differences between transdisciplinary and traditionally trained doctoral students: A comparison of publication patterns. *Plos One*, doi.org/10.1371/journal.pone.0189391

Keyton, J., Ford, D. J., & Smith, F. I. (2008). A mesolevel communicative model of collaboration. *Communication Theory, 18*(3), 376–406. doi:10.1111/j.1468-2885.2008.00327.x

Lemieux-Charles, L., & McGuire, W. L. (2006). What do we know about health care team effectiveness? A review of the literature. *Medical Care Research and Review, 63*(3), 263–300. doi:10.1177/1077558706287003

Littlechild, B., & Smith, R. (2013). *A handbook for interprofessional practice in the human services.* doi:10.4324/9781315833620

Mattessich, P.W., & Monsey B. R. (1992) *Collaboration: What Makes It Work.* A Review of Research Literature on Factors Influencing Successful Collaboration. St. Paul, MN: Amherst Wilder Foundation

Miller, R. C. (2017). Interdisciplinarity: Its meaning and consequences. *Oxford Research Enclyclopedia of International Studies* (online). doi:10.1093/acrefore/9780190846626.013.92. Retrieved from https://oxfordre.com/internationalstudies/view/10.1093/acrefore/9780190846626.001.0001/acrefore-9780190846626-e-92

Newell, W. H. (2007). Distinctive challenges of library-based interdisciplinary research and writing: A guide. *Issues in Integrative Studies, 25*, 28–110.

Podean, M. I., Benta, D., & Rusu, L. (2011). About creativity in collaborative systems - Why it matters and how it can be supported. *Proceedings of the International Conference on E-Business*, 151–154. doi:10.5220/0003524501510154

Schöttle, A., Haghsheno, S., & Gehbauer, F. (2014). Defining cooperation and collaboration in the context of lean construction – Teaching lean construction. Oslo, Norway: Conference Proceedings IGLC-22. Retrieved from https://pdfs.semanticscholar.org/bc5a/b6892330e4aa01f11e4902d2eeba013e6e97.pdf

Schrage, M. (1995). *No more teams!: Mastering the dynamics of creative collaboration.* New York, NY: Currency Doubleday.

Shelbourn, M., Bouchlaghem, N., Anumba, C., & Carrillo, P. (2007). Planning and implementation of effective collaboration in construction projects. *Construction Innovation, 7*(4), 357–377. doi:10.1108/14714170710780101

Stone J. (2009). *Interprofessional collaborative practice: Definitions and terminology.* Canberra, Australia: Australian Capital Territory Health.

Thomas, S. E., & Leonard, A. E. (2014). Interdisciplinary librarians: Self-reported non-LIS scholarship and creative work. *Library Management, 35*(8/9), 547–557. doi:10.1108/LM-02-2014-0030

Thomson, A. M., & Perry, J. L. (2006, November 09). Collaboration processes: Inside the black box. Retrieved from https://onlinelibrary.wiley.com/doi/full/10.1111/j.1540-6210.2006.00663.x

Thomson, A. M., Perry, J. L., & Miller, T. K. (2007). Conceptualizing and measuring collaboration. *Journal of Public Administration Research and Theory, 19*(1), 23–56. doi:10.1093/jopart/mum036

Wilkes, S. E., & Miodownik, M. A. (2018). Materials library collections as tools for interdisciplinary research. *Interdisciplinary Science Reviews, 43*(1), 3–23, doi:10.1080/03080188.2018.1435450

World Health Organization. (2015, December 21). Framework for action on interprofessional education and collaborative practice. Retrieved from https://www.who.int/hrh/resources/framework_action/en/

4

COMMUNITIES AND COMMUNITY ENGAGEMENT

Henry R. Cunningham

There are many questions regarding the myriad number of complex issues that are of concern to communities, both urban and rural. Many of these communities, particularly urban, experienced decline due to deindustrialization and globalization, resulting in the loss of jobs (Harkavy & Zuckerman, 1999; Taylor & Luter, 2013). Many of the manufacturing jobs on which communities depended disappeared and the new jobs created required skills that laborers did not possess, as a knowledge-based economy became more dominant (Hackworth, 2007). The loss of jobs created several challenges for communities, chief among them, that of unemployment (Initiative for a Competitive Inner City, 2011). This resulted in other social issues such as poor schools, blighted neighborhoods, general poverty (Taylor & Luter, 2013), and increased crime rates (Harkavy & Zuckerman, 1999).

Parker et al. (2018) from the Pew Research Center enforced this point regarding the many problems facing both rural and urban communities. According to a study conducted, they indicated some problems are common across all communities, while others are unique to either urban or rural communities. The issue of drug addiction is reported to be common among both urban and rural communities, with 50% and 46%, respectively, of surveyed respondents in their study, having this view. In the urban communities, other issues cited by residents who were part of the study include affordable housing, poverty, crime, and the quality of public schools. The study also highlighted that rural residents are more concerned about the availability of jobs and a lack of access to public transportation. Access to health care also seems to be a concern for rural communities as two-thirds of residents claimed it was either a major or a minor issue for them.

This chapter will explore how communities addressed many of the issues that arose by partnering with institutions such as colleges and universities and libraries among others. It will explore the nature of these partnerships and collaborations, particularly as they relate to university-community partnerships, focusing on their importance and challenges encountered. The chapter will deal with important aspects of the primary motivation behind the collaboration and the mutual benefits for both communities and the partnering institution.

Boyer (1996), former president of the Carnegie Foundation for Teaching and Learning, noted that social issues abound in communities and can only be addressed through partnerships and collaboration of various entities. He said, "the academy must become a more vigorous partner in the search for answers to our most pressing social, civic, economic, and moral problems" (p. 11). For higher education, the objective is to enhance the town-gown relationships between the institution and community through teaching, research, and service in what has become to be known as community engagement.

Reasons for community engagement

There are many reasons why organizations come together to work collaboratively on projects. Because of the many social issues plaguing rural and urban communities, many have turned to institutions of higher learning, which bring with them expertise and resources that can help communities address these problems. For universities, the increased interest in knowledge transfer (Ostrander, 2004) as well as historical context, institutional mission, and the expectation from the community for them to address critical community issues (Bringle & Hatcher, 2002) prompted them to partner with their communities. In a study conducted by Vaterlaus et al. (2016), they reported that university faculty surveyed reported that the purpose of their partnership with community entities was to address university needs that could be addressed through partnerships. These needs included existing audiences, locations to hold events and contribution of other resources. The mutual benefit associated with partnership is a driving force for its creation as in the case of Metropolitan State University in Minnesota and the Saint Paul Community Library. Both needed a library and through collaboration one was constructed to address the need of the University and the community (Shumer et al., 2009).

Institutions such as Metropolitan State University are anchor institutions in their respective communities. These universities are in a unique position to partner with community stakeholders to address the issues that are of concern. As anchors, they are place-based engines that play key roles in local economies (Slavek, 2019; Perry & Menendez, 2011), are immobile, and have a connection to their communities (Harkavy & Zuckerman, 1999). Because of their immobility they are stable and provide permanence to the community, which enables them to be involved in community revitalization (Harkavy & Hodges, 2012). In addition, as institutions of higher learning, they bring with them a wealth of resources in faculty and student expertise (Taylor & Luter, 2013). Having this much resources at their disposal prompted Harkavy and Hodges (2012) to argue that institutions of higher learning have a moral and ethical responsibility to the wellbeing of their communities.

There are several examples of anchor institutions engaging with their communities to address pressing issues. In the United States, Johns Hopkins University created the East Baltimore Redevelopment, Inc. where it was attempting to address the issues of poverty, drugs, crime, and a high vacancy rate in the neighborhood. The University of Pennsylvania spent approximately $100 million partnering with the Pennsylvania Minority Business Center to assist small businesses to do business with the University (Initiative for a Competitive Inner City, 2011). The University of Louisville likewise, partnered with the west Louisville community to create the Signature Partnership Initiative, which was developed to address issues of unemployment, health disparities, educational attainment, and social services in the community (Cunningham et al., 2015; Cunningham & Lewis, 2010). This initiative created opportunities for community-engaged teaching, research, and service to address community identified needs. It utilized a conceptual framework involving academic units and some administrative units partnering with the west Louisville community. This framework provides a more comprehensive approach to addressing the issues in the community (Carriere, 2008; Cunningham et al., 2009; Gifford et al., 2005). Other institutions took on statewide projects, covering a larger geographical area. Arizona State University was involved with statewide issues through the "New American University", Initiative, on such projects as immigration and water use (Weerts, 2011). In the United Kingdom, the DigitalCity Initiative in Teesside in partnership with Teesside University boosted employment with the creation of technology businesses and new jobs. This resulted in a major economic boom for the community (Payne, 2017).

The nature of partnerships in community engagement

In addition to addressing community needs these partnerships must ensure that there is common ground among the partners. This includes having shared values (Initiative for a Competitive City, 2011), goals, and objectives that make the partnership compatible (Vaterlaus et al., 2016), a clear understanding of each other's wants, needs, and values (Curwood et al., 2011) and having "shared vision, practices and experiences" (Fletcher et al., 2017, p. 86). The presence of these factors is important to ensure a viable partnership is developed and sustained over time.

Several other elements must be in place for partnerships to start, grow, and blossom. This involves having a partnership model that works for both parties. Partnership models vary depending on the nature of the partnership and the organizations involved. Bryan and Henry (2012) developed a seven-stage model of developing school-family-community partnerships, which works well when the school, family, and community partners are collaborating. The seven stages of the model include (a) preparing to partner, (b) assessing needs and strengths, (c) coming together, (d) creating shared vision and plan, (e) taking action, (f) evaluating and celebrating success, and (g) maintain momentum. They argue that this model involves "democratic collaboration, empowerment, social justice, and a strengths focus" (p. 411) that promotes healthy collaboration between and among partners.

Hudson and Hardy (2002) presented a model that seems to work well for university-community partnership. They identified six principles of university-community partnerships: (a) acknowledgment of the need for partnership; (b) clarity and realism of purpose; (c) commitment; (d) development and maintenance of trust; (e) establishment of clear and robust partnership arrangements; (f) monitoring, review, and organizational learning. These principles are important for university-community partnerships because they establish the expectation for the collaborative effort to be successful. For instance, acknowledging the need for partnership is an indication from both parties that there is an issue of concern to both that needs to be addressed. Archur-Kuhn and Grant (2014), using these principles in a university-community partnership, noted that it created a "picture perfect" (p. 43) project for them.

For university-community partnerships to be successful, they must also reflect certain factors that are essential for collaboration. A few of these include (a) mutual respect and trust, (b) clear and common goals and vision, (c) dialogue and communication, (d) developing and nurturing relationships, (e) involvement, and (f) prioritizing the community and maintaining a community focus (Carlton et al., 2009). These factors play a critical role in guiding the direction of the partnership and ensuring success, and all elements are necessary for a viable collaboration. For instance, it is important that both parties respect each other and what is brought to the partnership. If there is an absence of mutuality, the likelihood that partners will be able to work together becomes more challenging. Likewise, they need to learn to trust each other as this strengthens the interactions (Suarez-Balcazar et al., 2005).

There are other models for developing and sustaining university-community partnerships including the Suarez-Balcazar et al. (2005) model, which provides a framework for such collaboration. These university-community partnerships models all have elements of successful traits. Therefore, partners must determine which model is most appropriate for them based on who they are and the nature of their partnership.

Different levels of community engagement

Community engagement is a continuum, meaning it may look different and be at varying stages based on the partners, the project, and the length of the partnership. In many cases the collaboration may start as an outreach activity, which is defined here as providing direct services, time, or resources to benefit a community or its institutions. Outreach is an easy first step in the collaboration but overtime as the partnership blossoms, community engagement may reach a higher level on the continuum and become more in-depth. Figure 4.1, modified by the authors from the International Association for Public Participation, provides the different levels of involvement in community engagement.

Increasing Level of Community Involvement, Impact, Trust, and Communication Flow

Some Community Involvement	More Community Involvement	Better Community Involvement	Community Involvement	Strong Bidirectional Relationship
Communication flows from one to the other, to inform	Communication flows to the community and then back, answer seeking	Communication flows both ways, participatory form of communication	Communication flow is bidirectional	Final decision making is at community level
Provides community with information		Involves more participation with community on issues	Forms partnerships with community on each aspect of project from development to solution	Entities have formed strong partnership structures
Entities co-exist	Gets information of feedback from the community			
Outcomes: Optimally, establishes communication channels and channels for outreach	Entities share information	Entities cooperate with each other	Entities form bidirectional communication channels	Outcomes: Broader health outcomes affecting broader community. Strong bidirectional trust built.
	Outcomes: Develops connections	Outcomes: Visibility of partnership established with increased cooperation	Outcomes: Partnership building, trust building	

FIGURE 4.1   Community engagement continuum.

Note: Reference modified by the authors from the International Association for Public Participation (Clinical Translational Science Awards Consortium Committee Task Force, 2011)

Source: Publicly Financed Document, no Permission Needed

This higher level of engagement includes joint decision-making, where universities and community partners have equal authority and responsibility in the partnership. A common aspect of engagement at this level is engaged-teaching and engaged-scholarship. At this, stage university faculty partners and community stakeholders together decide on teaching and research initiatives that are beneficial to students, the faculty, and the community.

Benefits of community engagement

When partnerships and collaboration occur, they bring many benefits to all parties involved. In the case of community engagement, both the university and community serve to benefit. For the university, this includes faculty, students, and the institution itself. Institutions of higher learning are provided opportunities to augment the application of scholarship (Williamson et al., 2017) and enhance understanding of their area of study (Klein et al., 2011). In addition, colleges and universities serve to benefit in other ways as collaborations build support and public advocacy for the institution within the community. It may also increase donor support and reinforce its place as a major contributor to the public good (Beere et al., 2011). For many in the community, institutions of higher learning are seen as an impenetrable space that is not accessible to them. Community collaborations provide an avenue for the community to access the university – its faculty, students, and other resources (Carriere, 2008).

Klein et al. (2011), in describing case studies of university-community partnerships, listed several benefits for faculty, including enhanced awareness and understanding of their content area, training opportunities for researchers, and "meaningful teaching and research" (p. 431). Collaborating with community partners on various projects provides faculty opportunities for research or new focus of research that they may never have pursued based on the opportunities afforded to them from the partnership. A Tufts University and Campus Compact publication, from a collective initiative of representatives of research universities and Campus Compact (2012), noted the work of Sandmann (2003), where she declared in an address to the National Extension Director/Administrator Conference that faculty who are engaged with the community also serve to benefit from the collaboration which cuts across teaching, research, and service. Community-engaged scholarship, which is defined as a form of scholarship derived from teaching, research, service, and creative activity that directly benefits the community and is consistent with university and unit missions, affords faculty to work on interdisciplinary and transdisciplinary projects, including colleagues from other academic units as they work collaboratively to address an issue from multiple perspectives – a practice that is also supported by Cunningham et al. (2009) and Sandmann (2003). According to Williamson et al. (2017), faculty members involved in community-engaged scholarship learn a new appreciation for translational research.

There are many benefits for students who engage with the community as part of their academic requirements, done primarily through courses. Community-based learning courses, also known as service-learning courses, allow students to apply course concepts to real-life issues in the community, where they engage in service that benefits the community. The benefits associated with community-based learning courses for students are well researched. Some benefits include improved academic performance (Markus et al., 1993); a greater likelihood of obtaining a college degree (Lockman & Pelco, 2013); a sense of civic responsibility (Astin & Sax, 1998); cultural awareness (Bloom, 2008; Borden, 2007); transformational learning, understanding oneself and relationship to social justice issues and practical skills applicable to the work place (Richards, 1996), to name a few. Warren (2012) suggested from a study he conducted, that service-learning also has a positive effect on student learning outcomes.

The benefits to communities from university collaborations are many and varied as institutions of higher learning lend their expertise and other resources to work on common goals and to come up with solutions to address the complex issues facing communities (Gronksi & Pigg, 2000). Benefits from the collaboration include such areas as building community capacity (Community Partner Summit Group, 2010), capacity building for community agency for research and evaluation, validation of existing efforts, and enhancing existing programs (Dugery & Knolwes, 2003). Williamson et al. (2017) also argued that university-community partnerships provide credibility to community organizations. They also stated that for community partners, collaborating with university faculty on research projects allow them to gain information that change the way they normally do things, utilizing more effective and efficient practices. In presenting several case studies of university-community partnerships, Klein et al. (2011) notes several benefits of the collaboration for community partners. In a social justice project with the University of Wisconsin, they stated some benefits included increased capacity for building relationships, increased visibility for the community and further access to the university. These partnerships may also help communities to find their voice and document their experiences (Bolin & Stanford, 1998; Kelland, 2016).

The concept of community engagement is beneficial to all parties involved. For faculty and students, it enhances teaching, learning, and research as new areas are explored in collaboration with community partners. For community partners, the wealth of expertise and other resources that institutions of higher learning bring with them is important in finding solutions to complex issues. Through these collaborations, much can be accomplished in a manner that benefits all. These benefits are not only applicable to university-community partnerships but to other partnerships as well, as may be between the community and health-care institutions, libraries, city and state governments, the private sector and other entities.

Challenges of community engagement

While these collaborative partnerships are often times successful and serve all involved, they sometimes bring with them challenges. Strier (2010) listed many of the challenges encountered in university-community partnerships. One major challenge is the unequal source of power that exists between universities and the community, whereby institutions of higher learning tend to wield more authority in such collaborations. Others challenges include bureaucratic constraints, poor planning and implementation, mistrust, competition for resources (Gray, 2004), ownership, funding, and lack of sustainability (Altman, 2005); cultural tensions (Carriere, 2008; Curwood et al., 2011); and differences between campuses and communities, cooperation and compromise (Beere et al., 2011); leadership change either within the university or community agency (Carriere, 2008). Scheduling and time commitment are also challenges as the university semester system is a short-term commitment to problems that are more long-term and require more time to address (Williamson et al., 2002). Also, sometimes when working in the community, it is difficult to determine who is the legitimate voice that speaks on behalf of the community when the group is unstructured and there is no clear leader (Ross et al., 2010). Such a situation can lead to mixed messages as a representative voice is missing.

These challenges can have negative impact on community engagement; therefore, partners must be cognizant of possible obstacles that may arise during collaborative efforts and take steps to address them. This requires adequate preparation before embarking on partnership, which includes being knowledgeable about the partner and potential pitfalls that may be encountered. It is important to know how your goals for the project aligned with the goals of your partner and the roles and responsibilities of all stakeholders. Challenges exist because individuals are different and may not always recognize how their differences can possibly influence a partnership. While these challenges exist and can negatively affect partnerships across the spectrum, the benefits derived may outweigh them.

Conclusion

Community engagement is dynamic and complex because of all that is involved; the purpose of the engagement, the primary motivation behind the collaboration, the multiple partners and what they can contribute to the effort, the nature of the issue at hand, the role of the partners, and unexpected developments that may arise, among others. While there are many challenges associated with community engagement, there are many benefits for all involved in the partnership. In the case of university-community partnerships, there are benefits for faculty teaching and research access to community expertise. For students, there are many benefits to their academic, social, and cultural growth. The institution from which faculty and students come serves to benefit as well, as does community partners with whom they are collaborating. Collaborative efforts serve everyone and are mutually beneficial, thus worth pursuing. Through community engagement, it is possible to address many societal issues. This collaborative effort may be advantageous for other institutions such as libraries and health-care facilities, including hospitals to pursue with their neighboring communities to address identified needs.

References

Altman, D. (2005). Communities, governments and AIDS: Making partnerships work. In P. Aggleton, P. Davies, & G. Hart (Eds.), *Aids, sexuality and risk* (pp. 109–117). London, England: Taylor & Francis.

Archur-Kuhn, B., & Grant, J. (2014). Challenging contextual factors in university-community partnerships. *Journal of Community Engagement and Scholarship, 7*(2), 40–49.

Astin, A. W., & Sax, L. J. (1998). How undergraduates are affected by service participation. *Journal of College Student Development, 39*(3), 251–263.

Beere, C. A., Votruba, J. C., & Wells, G. W. (2011). *Becoming an engaged campus: A practical guide for institutionalizing public engagement.* San Francisco, CA: Jossey Bass.

Bloom, M. (2008). From the classroom to the community: Building cultural awareness in first semester Spanish. *Language, Culture, and Curriculum, 21*(2), 103–119.

Bolin, R., & Stanford, L. (1998). The Northridge earthquake: Community-based approaches to unmet recovery needs. *Disasters, 22*(1), 21–28. doi.org/10.1111/1467-7717.00073

Borden, A.W. (2007). The impact of service-learning on ethnocentrism in an intercultural communication course. *Journal of Experiential Education, 30*(2), 171–183.

Boyer, E. L. (1996). The scholarship of engagement. *Journal of Public Service and Outreach, 1*(1), 11–20.

Bringle, R. G., & Hatcher, J. A. (2002). Campus-community partnerships: The terms of engagement. *Journal of Social Issues, 58*(3), 503–516.

Bryan, J., & Henry, L. (2012). A model for building school-family-community partnerships: Principles and process. *Journal of Counseling and Development, 90,* 408–420. doi:10.1002/j.1556-6676.2012.00052.x

Carlton, E. L., Whiting, J. B., Bradford, K., Dyk, P. H., & Vail, A. (2009). Defining factors of successful university-community collaborations: An exploration of one healthy marriage project. *Family Relations Interdisciplinary Journal of Applied Family Studies, 58*(1), 28–40. doi:10.1111/j.1741-3729.2008.00532.x

Carriere, A. (2008). Community engagement through partnerships – A primer. *Metropolitan Universities, 19*(1), 84–100.

Clinical and Translational Science Awards Consortium Community Engagement Key Function Committee Task Force on the Principles of Community Engagement. (2011). *Principles of community engagement* (2nd ed.). Retrieved from https://www.atsdr.cdc.gov/communityengagement/pdf/PCE_Report_508_FINAL.pdf

Community Partner Summit Group. (2010). Achieving the promise of community-higher education partnerships: Community partners get organized. In H. E. Fitzgerald, C. Burack, & S. D. Seifer (Eds.), *Handbook of engaged scholarship: Contemporary landscapes, future directions* (2nd ed., pp. 201–221). East Lansing: Michigan State University Press.

Cunningham, H. R., Hines-Martin, V., & Hall, D. (2015). The signature partnership initiative: A university-community partnership initiative. *The International Journal of Community Diversity, 15*(4), 17–31.

Cunningham, H. R., Kennedy, J., Clark, T., Walker, K. L., Hart, J. L., Hutti, M. H., … Todd, D. D. (2009). Providing healthcare: An interdisciplinary international service-learning approach. In M. Moore & P. L. Lin (Eds.), *Service-learning in higher education: Paradigms and challenges* (pp. 357–372). Indianapolis, IN: University of Indianapolis Press.

Cunningham, H. R., & Lewis, S. (2010). Enhancing public school education: A collaborative partnership for school resiliency. *Metropolitan Universities, 20*(3), 25–33.

Curwood SE, Munger F, Mitchell T, Mackergan M Farrar A (2011) Building effective community-university partnerships: Are universities truly ready. Michigan Journal of community service learning, 17(2), 15–26.

Dugery, J., & Knolwes, J. (2003). *University + community research partnerships: A new approach.* Charlottesville, VA: Pew Partnership for Civic Change.

Fletcher, F., Hibbert, A., Hammer, B., & Ladouceur, S. (2017). Beyond collaboration: Principles and indicators of authentic relationship development in CBPR. *Journal of Community Engagement and Scholarship, 9*(2), 81–91.

Gifford, D., Strenecky, B. J., & Cunningham, H. R. (2005). International service-learning successfully engaging adult students. *Metropolitan Universities, 16*(2), 53–62.

Gray, B. (2004). Strong opposition: Frame-based resistance to collaboration. *Journal of Community and Applied Psychology, 14,* 166–176. doi:10.1002/casp.773

Gronksi, R., & Pigg, K. (2000). University and community collaboration. *American Behavioral Scientist, 43,* 781–793.

Hackworth, J. R. (2007). The neoliberal city: Governance ideology, and development in America urbanism. Ithaca, NY: Cornell University Press.

Harkavy, I., & Hodges, R. A. (2012). Democratic devolution: How America's colleges and universities can strengthen their communities. Netter Center for Community Partnerships, University of Pennsylvania.

Harkavy, I., & Zuckerman, H. (1999). *Eds and meds: Cities' hidden assets.* Washington, DC: Center on Urban and Metropolitan Policy, The Brookings Institute.

Hudson, B., & Hardy, B. (2002). What is a "successful" partnership and how can it be measured? In C. Glendinnning, M. Powell, & Rummery, K. (Eds.), *Partnerships, new labour and the governance of welfare* (pp. 51–66). Bristol, England: The Policy Press.

Initiative for a Competitive Inner City. (2011). Inner city insights: Anchor institutions and urban economic development. *Inner City Insights Finding, 1*(2), 1–9.

Kelland, L. (2016). Digital community engagement across the divides. *history@work*. National Council on Public History. https://ncph.org/history-at-work/digital-community-engagement-across-the-divides/

Klein, P. K., Fatima, M., Mcewen, L., Moser, S. C., Schmidt, D., & Zupan, S. (2011). Dismantling the ivory tower: Engaging geographers in university–community partnerships. *Journal of Geography in Higher Education, 35*(3), 425–444. doi:10.1080/03098265.2011.576337

Lockman, K. S., & Pelco, L. E. (2013). The relationship between service-learning and degree completion. *Michigan Journal of Community Service Learning, 20*(1), 18–30.

Markus, G. B., Howard, J. P., & King, D. C. (1993). Integrating community service and classroom instruction enhances learning: Results from an experiment. *Educational Evaluation and Policy Analysis, 15*(4), 410–419.

Ostrander, S. A. (2004). Democracy, civic participation, and the university: A comparative study of civic engagement on five campuses. *Nonprofit and Voluntary Sector Quarterly, 33*(1), 74–93. doi:10.1177/0899764003260588

Parker, K., Horowitz, J. M., Brown, A., Fry, R., Cohn, D., & Igielnik, R. (2018). What unites and divides urban, suburban and rural communities. Retrieved from Pew Research Center, Social and Demographic Trends Website: https://www.pewsocialtrends.org/2018/05/22/what-unites-and-divides-urban-suburban-and-rural-communities/

Payne, D. (2017, April 24). Maximizing the role of the UK universities as "anchor institutions". Nature jobs Blog post. Retrieved from http://blogs.nature.com/naturejobs/2017/04/24/maximising-the-role-of-uk-universities-as-anchor-institutions/

Perry, D., & Menendez, C. (2011). The impact of institutions of higher education on urban and metropolitan areas: Assessment of the coalition of urban and metropolitan universities. Retrieved from Community-Wealth.Org Website: https://community-wealth.org/content/impact-institutions-higher-education-urban-and-metropolitan-areas-assessment-coalition-urban

Richards, R. W. (1996). *Building partnerships: Educating health professionals for the communities they serve.* San Francisco, CA: Jossey Bass.

Ross, L. F., Loup, A., Nelson, R. M., Botkin, J. R., Kost, R., Smith Jr., G. R., & Gehlert, S. (2010). The challenges of collaboration for academic and community partners in a research partnership: Points to consider. *Journal of Empiraical Research on Human and Research Ethics, 5*(1), 19–31. doi:10.1525/jer.2010.5.1.19

Sandmann, L. (2003, February). *When doing good is not good enough. Good to great: The scholarship of engagement.* Address to the National Extension Director/Administrator Conference, Fort Lauderdale, Florida.

Shumer, R., Shumer, S., Ryan, R., Brooks, J., Cejudo, M. A. R., & DuPaul, K. (2009). Metropolitan state university: Connecting with community through a university-community library partnership. In T. Kelshaw, F. Lazarus, J. Miner, & Associates (Ed.), *Partnership, for service-learning: Impacts on communities and students* (pp. 75–102). San Francisco, CA: Jossey Bass.

Slavek, E. (2019). The transformative power of anchor institutions. *Metropolitan Universities, 30*(1), 3–4. doi:10.18060/22919

Strier, R. (2010). The construction of university-community partnerships: entangled perspective. High Educ 62, 81–97 (2011). https://doi.org/10.1007/s10734-010-9367-x

Suarez-Balcazar Y., Harper, G. W., & Lewis, R. (2005). An interactive and contextual model of community-university collaborations for research and action. *Health Education and Behavior, 32*(1), 84–101. doi:10.1177/1090198104269512

Taylor, H. L., & Luter, G. (2013). Anchor institutions: An interpretive review essay. University of Buffalo. Anchor Institutions Task Force.

Tufts University & Campus Compact. (2012). New times demand new scholarship I: Research universities and civic engagement: A leadership agenda. *Journal of Higher Education Outreach and Engagement, 16*(4), 235–269.

Vaterlaus, J. M., Skygrand, L., Higginbotham, B. J., & Bradford, K. (2016). Sustaining university-community partnerships in providing relationship education. *Journal of Community Engagement and Scholarship, 9*(2), 34–40. Retrieved from http://jces.ua.edu/wp-content/uploads/2017/04/04_JCES-9.2-Sustaining-University-Community-Partnerships.pdf

Warren, J. L. (2012). Does service-learning increase student learning?: A meta-analysis. *Michigan Journal of Community Service Learning, 18*(2), 56–61.

Weerts, D. J. (2011). "If only we told our story better…': Re-envisioning state-university relations through the Lens of Public Engagement." WISCAPE Viewpoints. Madison, WI: University of Wisconsin–Madison, Wisconsin Center for the Advancement of Postsecondary Education (WISCAPE). Retrieved from https://eric.ed.gov/?id=ED518998

Williamson, H. J., Young, B., Murray, N., Burton, D. L., Lubotsky, L., Massey, O.T., & Baldwin, J. A. (2016). Community-university partnerships for research and practice: Application of an interactive and contextual model of collaboration. Journal of Higher Education Outreach and Engagement, 20(2), 55–84.

PART II
Project exemplars

SECTION A
Information literacy

5

INTRODUCTION

Fannie M. Cox

In this book several chapters in Part II – Project Exemplars –discuss how librarians are moving the profession of Librarianship forward, through outreach, collaborations, and partnerships. These chapters represent transformation of how "direct aid to users of the library" has not changed, but has expanded beyond physicality. Librarians are staying true to the core of Librarianship regardless of library type, by collaborating with other organizations to use and maximize existing assets in innovative ways to broaden access to those in need. The described processes and lessons-learned have application for low-, middle-, and high-resource settings and a variety of populations significantly impacted by many barriers such as environmental factors, language, location/distance, access, cost, housing, health, and medical.

Within these chapters, librarians provide insight into their involvement in the community, with curriculum and technology support, collection development, Information Literacy (IL) and instructional design, irrespective of culture, socioeconomic, educational level, and location that will illuminate the philosophy and perspectives that serve as a foundation for libraries and librarians as key players in collaborations to enhance health and quality of life. They met the user where they were, and through collaboration their information needs were met. Although challenges did arise, they provided lessons-learned and success was ultimately achieved.

Libraries have always been around. As place in communities and the academy, it is the anchor. During times of crisis – while the digital divide continues to exist, homelessness is still problematic, other societal ills arise, or become a community problem – libraries will then continue to be the "safe place" to use computers, find information, and get assistance.

As more and more organizations and educational institutions realize and acknowledge the presence and take into account, its reach in the community only will the impact of both academic and public libraries be fully understood. The following chapters of exemplars only scratch the surface of how impactful libraries are when collaboration, partnerships, and Community Engagement are used as tools to bring together each other's resources, assets, and knowledge to bring about change for the good of those who needed assistance.

6

BUILDING WELLNESS PARTNERSHIPS IN GRADUATE LIBRARY AND INFORMATION SCIENCE (LIS) EDUCATION

Loriene Roy, Yan Zhang, and Nora Rose

Introduction: graduate Library and Information Science (LIS) education and service learning

Students in graduate programs preparing for careers in the information professions have long been involved in direct work with service communities through their formal and informal coursework (Roy, 2009). Such arrangements are dependent on establishing and maintaining partnerships outside of the classroom. Students often have many opportunities to initiate, test, and develop partnerships in their graduate education. They might accomplish this through their employment and volunteer work, but also within courses. Within courses, students may seek out community partners to test ideas, practice and acquire skills, and establish connections that might lead to future employment. Community partners gain access to willing volunteers and often to cutting edge practice, skills, and resources.

This section illustrates three partnerships that were established to provide opportunities for students to connect with community groups to explore aspects of health literacy. Each partnership required diligent planning and was time dated, lasting, in general, over the course of a 16-week semester. Details are provided on the learning objects such as websites, videos, pathfinders, and LibGuides the students created through these partnerships. This section will discuss challenges encountered and conclude with recommendations for educators, clients, and students.

Partnership one: LIS students and the ALA President's workplace wellness initiative

Founded in 1876 and with a current membership of some 58,000, the American Library Association (ALA) is the oldest and largest professional library association in the world (American Library Association, 2019). Each year the membership elects an individual to serve as president-elect. Their year as president-elect extends from the end of the ALA annual conference, usually held in late June, until the closing of the next ALA annual conference. During the president-elect year, they generally work with an advisory board to advance the issues they select to highlight.

The 2007–2008 ALA President chose workplace wellness as one of her presidential initiatives (Roy, 2008). The President was concerned that library workers, while attentive to the needs of their patrons, were not mindful of their own needs, especially their own personal health. Her view of workplace wellness focused on how library workers might find balance in multiple aspects of their life that, ultimately, would impact their ability to also be fulfilled in their work. To address this issue, one of her former students designed a website that provided resources including documents to assist ALA members to stay healthy when attending conferences.

Seven years later, a group of ALA Emerging Leaders revised the workplace wellness website. A new ALA President chose to once again support ALA members through attention on workplace wellness. While the new President's Advisory Board provided advice, the work fell once again in the lap of a School of Information (iSchool) graduate student to redesign the website. The selected student volunteered to conduct this work through an elective individual studies course. She reviewed the 2007–2008 workplace wellness website, completed Institutional Review Board (IRB) human subjects research training, conducted a literature review, and collaborated with the ALA President's Advisory Board's Wellness Team to expand and enrich content on the website. New content addressed topics including financial and social wellness. With a home page featuring the faces of ALA members, content was presented on eight aspects of personal wellness: emotional, environmental, financial, intellectual, occupational, physical, spiritual, and social. The launch was covered in a press release from ALA as well as in an article in the newsletter, *Library Worklife* (Morales, 2018; ALA President, 2018).

Partnership two: LIS students and Health Alliance for Austin Musicians (HAAM)

In Austin, Texas, a city known as the Live Music Capitol of the World, organizations have been founded to assist musicians with their medical needs. One such organization is Health Alliance for Austin Musicians (HAAM). Members of HAAM include musicians, disc jockeys, and music teachers residing in Travis County, Texas. HAAM staff assist HAAM members in navigating the marketplace of insurance providers available through the Affordable Care Act. In addition, HAAM members can take advantage of other HAAM services such as a voucher for dental services, a vision test and discounted eyewear, hearing testing and discounted customized ear plugs, and discounts for services such as massage, acupuncture, and chiropractic (HAAM, 2019).

Students in two graduate classes partnered with HAAM to assist in advancing health literacy among HAAM members. Students in one class – the Library

Instruction and Information Literacy class – created videos to share HAAM's messages. The completed videos covered the topics of hearing health and HAAM services, health-care literacy, navigating insurance vocabulary, and an overview of HAAM services. Through their actions in creating products of use to a community organization and reflecting on their work, students engage in service-learning, satisfying the description of this pedagogical approach:

> Through high-quality service-learning, students perform activities that directly address human and community needs. In addition, students engage in critical reflection about what social responsibility means to them and how they will make socially responsible choices throughout all aspects of their lives.
>
> *(Jacoby & Associates, 2003, p. xvii)*

Students enrolled in the following semester "Consumer Health Informatics" class reviewed the HAAM website, interviewed a HAAM representative concerning their needs through emails, and created new sharable content. One example of such content was a flyer promoting HAAM members' awareness of hearing health.

Additionally, two students created an app (mockup) based on both learning theories and health behavior models to enhance musicians' knowledge of hearing health and promote the adoption of healthy behaviors.

Partnership three: LIS students and the Library of Congress Literacy Awards Advisory Board

In 2013, the Library of Congress launched the Library of Congress Literacy Awards with funding from Mr. David Rubenstein. There are three annual Library of Congress Literacy Awards and up to 15 best practice honorees recognized each year (Library of Congress, 2019).

Recipients of the David M. Rubenstein Prize included Reach Out and Read, Room to Read, First Book, WETA Reading Rockets, the Children's Literacy Initiative, and Reading is Fundamental. American Prize recipients included efforts with students and young readers such as 826 National, SMART, and United Through Reading, and the Parent-Child Home Program, the National Center for Families Learning, and New York City's East Side Community School.

In spring 2019, graduate students in a library instruction class created learning objects for members of the Library of Congress Literacy Awards Advisory Board. These consisted of pathfinders or text documents that provided an introduction to one of a number of topics related to literacy, an annotated bibliography of 15–25 sources, along with a two-page pathfinder that provides a strategy for locating relevant resources on the selected topic. Students also had the option to suggest a literacy topic that might be of interest to the Advisory Board. Students worked individually. Final pathfinders were completed mid-way through the semester.

In addition, students converted their pathfinders to LibGuides that were hosted in an educational sandbox provided by the LibGuide company, Springshare. The sandbox allowed students to share their LibGuides with each other and with students in other graduate programs that had access to the sandbox. The policies of using the sandbox did not permit students to share the LibGuides directly with their clients.

Included in the pathfinders was one created by a student on health literacy, defined as an individual's capacity to acquire, understand, and act appropriately on health information (US Department of Health and Human Services, n.d.). Health literacy spans a range of skills, from being able to converse comfortably with a doctor regarding a diagnosis to using math to understand the results of blood work. Health literacy can also encompass issues not directly related to an individual's health concerns. For example, health literacy can also include being able to confidently select a suitable health insurance plan. To realize more extensive health literacy, proponents in the United States typically advocate for the use of simpler language; improved access to and diffusion of health information; and more equitable, transparent communication between experts and the public.

The first aspect of the pathfinder's scope defined the parameters of health literacy: what it is, how it is implemented, and the challenges to achieving it. The second aspect of scope concentrated on the kinds of resources used to help promote and encourage health literacy. Taken together, the pathfinder sought to answer preliminary questions about health literacy as a practice. Questions users might ask on the topic are: What is health literacy? What are the challenges in increasing health literacy? How can I evaluate health literacy (either my own or that of my community)? How can I promote health literacy? What are some resources I can provide to others to strengthen health literacy?

The resources selected were scientifically reputable and, where possible, not-for-profit and free of advertisements. Similarly, the student made an effort to include resources that were free or easily accessible and written in plain language.

Challenges and lessons learned

Bishop et al. (2009) pointed out a weakness in involving students in service-learning:

> The discourse of service-learning sometimes limits its pedagogical implications by not considering bidirectional exchange in which both students and community members are learners. But learning cannot be an activity independent of learners' lives, experiences, and community. We suggest instead that students and community members work together to develop critical consciousness, democratic citizenship, and social justice.

Incorporating community-based partnerships within the graduate classroom brings challenges as well as opportunities. Students benefit from learning how to create products that have the potential for serving broad and varied audiences. Their contributions introduce community partners to the studies conducted and potential work products possible in information studies graduate programs. Community partners may benefit from having work completed that helps them accomplish their missions and extend their often small workforce. For faculty, these partnerships bring continuous change, enabling them to refresh their own learning.

Many of the challenges in these service-learning experiences are addressed in the need for continual communication and feedback. These challenges are transformed into recommendations in the final part of this section.

Recommendations for educators, clients, and students

This section presents three cases to illustrate how graduate students, guided by their faculty, can collaborate with professional groups in advancing knowledge of health literacy. These recommendations are offered for others based on these experiences.

In these partnerships, educators serve as the link between clients and students. Faculty often identify and recruit clients and translate client needs into assignments. Ideally, this recruitment takes place well in advance of the first day of class. Faculty work with the client to confirm communication protocol, ensuring that students have a means through which they can receive answers to their questions while respecting the client's time. Faculty write descriptions of assignments, create evaluation rubrics, assist students in acquiring the needed skills to create their health literacy learning objects, provide feedback, assess student work, and make sure that clients receive timely access to completed work. Faculty need to adjust their own schedules and that of their students to accommodate the clients' schedules. At the same time, they need to remind the client of the students' timelines and the academic schedule. Such schedules include due dates by which students submit work and faculty members evaluate student work so that faculty might submit final grades in accordance with university deadlines.

Recommendations for educators include the following:

- Incorporate both flexibility and structure
- Encourage and employ clear communication with students and clients
- Assist students in understanding the dynamics of successful group work
- Have a clear idea of what final work might look like while leaving students with the freedom and support to create unexpected yet successful end products
- Acquire a listening and witnessing approach to hearing student and client needs

Clients have served as the focal point of these efforts. Their needs define the purpose of the collaborative work as the educators and students translate them into tangible outcomes. Clients introduce their work settings and organizational missions and provide students with insights into employment. Their feedback informs the faculty on the usefulness of student work and, thus, assists faculty in continuously revising course assignments. Clients provide the narrative through which students can assess the impact of their work.

Recommendations for clients include the following:

- Clearly describe their goals for a successful partnership with educators and students
- Respond promptly to questions
- Review student work as it develops
- Provide feedback as needed
- Continue contact to describe the impact of the student work

Students are building foundational subject content for their future careers as well as a palette of technical skills. They are learning about the information professions, and testing and acquiring the skills needed in these service areas.

Recommendations for students include the following:

- Trust that their work will be completed and will satisfy the requirements of their assignment
- Be open to learning content and skills that extend beyond that of the written syllabus
- Communicate with their client as needed and share such communication with their faculty
- Be cognizant that clients have work schedules that might hamper their ability to respond on demand
- Illustrate the skills of a considerate and constructive team member
- Demonstrate initiative as well as accommodation

Conclusion

LIS faculty and their students can successfully develop partnerships with community organizations through providing service-learning opportunities within formal classes. While there are many challenges to faculty and students collaborating with community partners in course-related projects, the benefits outweigh the challenges encountered. Such opportunities assist students in acquiring marketable skills in teamwork while reflecting on their academic and personal skills. Community organizations benefit through welcoming students as peer contributors, gaining work that they might have difficulty accomplishing. Faculty benefit by seeing the impact of their service orientation on their communities and seeing the potential of what students are capable of creating.

References

ALA President unveils enriched ALA-APA workplace wellness website. (2018, July). *Library Worklife.* Retrieved from http://ala-apa.org/newsletter/2018/07/10/ala-president-unveils-enriched-ala-apa-workplace-wellness-website

American Library Association. (2019). *About ALA.* Retrieved from http://www.ala.org/aboutala/

Bishop, A., Bruce, B. C., & Jeong, S. (2009). Beyond service learning: Toward community schools and reflective community learners. In L. Roy, K. Jensen, & A. Meyers (Eds.), *Service learning: Linking library education and practice* (pp. 16–31). Chicago, IL: American Library Association.

HAAM. (2019). *About HAAM.* Retrieved from https://myhaam.org/our-story/

Jacoby, B., & Associates. (2003). *Building partnerships for service-learning.* San Francisco, CA: Jossey-Bass.

Library of Congress. (2019). *Literacy awards.* Retrieved from: https://www.loc.gov/item/prn-19-081/library-of-congress-announces-winners-of-2019-literacy-awards/2019-08-29/

Morales, M. (2018, July 9). *ALA President unveils enriched ALA-APA workplace wellness website.* Retrieved from http://ala.org/news/press-releases/2018/07/ala-president-enveils-enriched-ala-apa-workplace-wellness-website

Roy, L. (2008, June/July). Circle of wellness. *American Libraries, 39*(6), 8.

Roy, L. (2009). Supporting LIS education through practice: Highlights of an ALA presidential year. In L. Roy, K. Jensen, & A. Meyers (Eds.), *Service learning: Linking library education and practice* (pp. vii–xii). Chicago, IL: American Library Association.

US Department of Health and Human Services Office of Disease Prevention and Health Promotion. "Quick Guide to Health Literacy." (n.d.). Retrieved from https://www.cecentral.com/assets/9828/Needs_Health%20Literacy%20-%20Fact%20Sheet_%20Health%20Literacy%20and%20Health%20Outcomes.pdf

7

INFORMATION LITERACY AND THE UNDERGRADUATE CURRICULUM

Engaging faculty and enhancing student learning

Hugh Burkhart

Introduction

Introducing students to information literacy concepts in their first year of higher education is a common practice. The Association of College and Research Libraries defines information literacy (IL) as "the set of integrated abilities encompassing the reflective discovery of information, the understanding of how information is produced and valued, and the use of information in creating new knowledge and participating ethically in communities of learning" (American Library Association, 2015). It is manifested in research skills such as topic selection, locating and utilizing resources, and citing sources appropriately. Library literature supports the use of first-year experience courses as a way to incorporate IL into the general education curriculum (Dhawan & Chen, 2014). Moreover, "[w]riting-intensive courses may be the high-impact practice for which information literacy is most often an explored, articulated component" (Riehle & Weiner, 2013, p. 133). By extension, first-year writing (FYW) courses are an ideal way to ensure as many students as possible are introduced to IL skills early in their academic careers. For librarians to be part of such an effort, however, there must be a collaborative relationship with faculty to embed research instruction into the courses faculty teach (Johnson-Grau et al., 2016). Ideally, there should also be a course with student learning outcomes (SLOs) corresponding to IL skills. This case study explores how librarians at the University of San Diego (USD) developed a relationship with FYW and worked not only to build library instruction into FYW classes but also to strengthen ties with discipline faculty and university administrators to implement the most effective approach to library research instruction.

Institutional context

At the end of the 2016–2017 academic year, the instruction program at USD's Copley Library was at a low ebb. A report conducted by the Reference department showed that from 2013 to 2017, library instruction sessions for the academic departments had steadily declined, from 172 sessions in 2013–2014 to 121 sessions in 2016–2017, or a 30% decrease over a four-year period. Most of these were "one-shots," meaning they occurred once during the semester, as opposed to multiple library sessions throughout the duration of the course (Buchanan & McDonough, 2017). The majority were for undergraduate courses, with no emphasis on either upper or lower division classes. While there was no single cause to which the decline could be attributed, what was evident was that librarians had gone from reaching nearly 3,500 students in a year to fewer than 2,500.

A national, Roman Catholic university, USD has a student population of over 9,000, with nearly 6,000 undergraduates and over 2,000 graduate students. Copley Library serves the entire campus with the exception of USD's School of Law. The library operates under the traditional departmental liaison model to support more than 900 full-time and adjunct faculty: liaison librarians are responsible for collection development, instruction, and research assistance in their areas and work to build close relationships with faculty. Until 2016–2017, the instruction emphasis at Copley Library had been placed on subject liaisons responsible for cultivating the relationships with faculty vital to maintaining IL instruction.

Under the university's old undergraduate core curriculum, there was no formal IL requirement and no true FYW program. The old core writing requirement, Composition and Literature (ENGL 121), focused on the critical analysis of literary texts and did not have SLOs truly relevant to IL skills. When a librarian was asked to conduct a session for ENGL 121, the emphasis was typically on a general orientation to the library unrelated to any assignments. Although Goldman et al. (2016) point out, "Students who receive an orientation to library resources and services are more likely to seek needed research assistance with course papers, projects, and presentations" (p. 82), without having the session timed at point of need, librarians did not have a focus to which to tie their content. Dhawan and Chen (2014) also note that research reinforces the notion that "students benefit more from library instruction if it is related to a specific assignment" (p. 425). Librarians also lacked a mechanism to assess the students they reached. Other than the student evaluations of the library's two credit-bearing classes and student and library peer evaluations for workshops and select one-shots, the library had no evidence to assess instruction as a whole.

Finding collaborators

Opportunities for more targeted IL instruction emerged with the introduction of the University's new core curriculum in Fall 2017. In development since 2011 and approved in 2016, the revised core curriculum included IL as one of its competencies in accordance with the university's accrediting body, the Western Association of Schools and Colleges (WASC) Senior College and University Commission, which articulates core competencies in its standards for student performance at graduation in the *Handbook of Accreditation* (WASC, 2013). At the time of its implementation, IL was embedded in USD's core curriculum along with Critical Thinking (collectively named CTIL) in Historical Inquiry courses. Prior to the core's implementation, the initial Historical Inquiry classes were first approved by the CTIL Area Task Force, which had a dedicated place for one librarian before the implementation of the revised core. A librarian was also part of the original Core Curriculum Committee charged with drafting the core in consultation with the academic units. That said, while the new Historical Inquiry classes did mean IL was now formally embedded in the university curriculum, librarians felt this situation to be less than ideal. Given the range of classes involved, it would be difficult for the History subject librarian to conduct IL sessions in all relevant courses and handle instruction for History classes that did not have the embedded core requirement. Moreover, since these classes occurred at both the upper and lower division levels, a student could conceivably fulfill the CTIL core requirement after the first year of university. A student could very well make it through the first year without any library orientation at all. Research suggests that library instruction appears to be most effective when scaffolded across the curriculum with "clearly defined goals for students at every level of university study" (Bowles-Terry, 2012, p. 91). Evidence cited above also points to the value of students being introduced to library skills in the first year. The situation at USD conformed to neither of these ideals. Luckily, the new core did offer an additional opportunity for librarians to reach students.

With the adoption of the new core, the old Composition and Literature requirement gave way to FYW to fulfill "the core curriculum requirement for lower division Written Communication" (University of San Diego). This class is taken by students in either their first or second semester. With more than 1,200 incoming first-year students in Fall 2017, this compulsory class presented the perfect opportunity to make the maximum impact on introductory library instruction. Copley Library's Coordinator of Instruction assembled a small team of willing librarians and reached out to the new Writing Program Director about collaborating with FYW instructors.

Two of the class' SLOs provided the impetus to begin the conversation. Under the heading of *Sources and Evidence*, these outcomes state that:

> Students will:
>
> - Use credible sources to develop ideas and arguments that are
> - Effective within assigned disciplines and discourses
> - Cite sources accurately according to topic and style
>
> *(University of San Diego, 2017)*

The Coordinator of Instruction and another librarian met with the Writing Program Director and FYW instructors prior to the fall semester. While collaboration with librarians to provide research instruction certainly was not a requirement, instructors were encouraged to work with librarians to support research instruction connected to relevant class assignments. For those instructors unfamiliar with the services librarians could provide, a generalized handout was distributed in person and via email to describe lessons librarians might include in one or more sessions for a given class (see Figure 7.1). Next, an online FYW subject guide was created for instructors to include in their Blackboard pages and librarians to use to direct students to tips for developing search strategies, finding and evaluating print and online sources, and citing references appropriately (see Figure 7.2). Finally, librarians agreed on a small set of core skills on which to focus from section to section. These included the skills listed above as well as distinguishing between scholarly and non-scholarly sources. Librarians had to remain fluid in their approach because while the FYW learning outcomes were static, the content in a given section varied depending on the instructor. Instructors requesting a session with a librarian were asked to provide their syllabi and any connected research assignments in advance. The Writing Program Director ensured the librarians had the contact information for all the instructors and reinforced her support for this project.

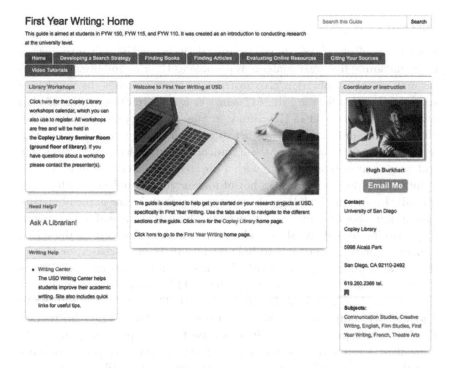

FIGURE 7.1   First year writing subject guide.

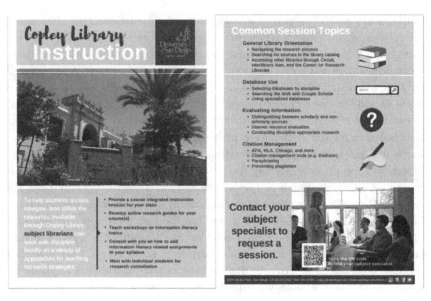

FIGURE 7.2 Library instruction handout.

Successes

Since the goal of this collaboration was relatively modest – to introduce as many incoming first-year students as possible to IL skills and library services through successful librarian/class instructor collaborations – the number of sessions scheduled for the Fall 2017 semester was heartening. Of the 27 class sections, librarians held 15 IL sessions, or 56% of the sections. The librarians also polled a number of students across multiple sections at the end of that semester. The vast majority of these students reported that the FYW section had been their only experience with a librarian in the classroom up to that point. While this is only a snapshot of undergraduate students, with an admittedly limited methodology, the response reinforced some of the librarians' assumptions about the number of students who previously had not been getting introduced to library skills and resources in their first year. In the spring semester, librarians were able to hold sessions in 18 of 30 classes, or 60% of the FYW sections. In total, nearly 500 first-year students received library instruction through this partnership alone. This translates to over 40% of first-year students admitted that academic year. The partnership with FYW undoubtedly contributed to the overall rise in the total library instruction number, which grew to 213, a 76% increase from the previous year. In all, more than 4,400 undergraduate and graduate students received IL instruction that year, a number never reached previously at the library and a vast improvement from the recent decline.

Continued success and new challenges

The following fall, the Coordinator of Instruction and the FYW library team again met with the Writing Program Director and instructors, this time to discuss successes from the previous year as well as solicit feedback from those who had collaborated with librarians. With the experience of a year-long partnership, librarians were confident in reaching out to individual instructors with whom they had collaborated to ask if they wished to work together again. Most did, and that fall, the partnerships grew further, with IL sessions from librarians occurring in 21 of 31 classes, 67% of the sections. That semester alone, the collaboration meant nearly 400 of 1,310 incoming first year students received library instruction in the fall. Librarians continued these outreach efforts in spring, hoping to capitalize on the success of the past three semesters. It was also time to evaluate the burgeoning program and any challenges faced.

The challenges of which librarians were already aware going into this project were mainly to do with organizational structure, both within the library and the writing program. At Copley Library, there is a Reference department, of which the Coordinator of Instruction is a member, but the department itself does not make decisions regarding library instruction. Up to this point, the Coordinator of Instruction's role was to chair instruction-related committees, oversee library credit-class scheduling, organize the student and faculty workshop series, and compile instruction statistics. Duties did not include a mandate to coordinate an instructional team for a given task or program. Now that there was a nascent program for first-year library instruction, the Coordinator had to find librarians willing to assist with the FYW teaching load. Two other librarians gladly took on these additional duties, but the Coordinator had to be mindful of their instruction commitments to their liaison areas and, in the case of one team member, a significant role in another department outside Reference. Without more teaching librarians on the team, issues with respect to scalability were anticipated, perhaps necessitating a restructuring within the library to meet the pedagogical and assessment needs required of more robust programming. One of the organizational challenges with respect to the Writing Program, on the other hand, was that instructors could vary from one semester to the next. Research in higher education shows that disciplines like English employ high numbers of adjunct faculty to meet teaching demands, especially at the introductory level (Morphew et al., 2017). The Writing Program at USD operates within the English department, which conforms to the trend of employing a large number of adjuncts. The department and the Writing Program share the same adjunct faculty, many of whom may teach courses other than FYW in a given semester. These adjuncts are often in temporary positions, and some are quite new to the university and, indeed, the teaching profession. Library literature notes the importance of relationships with adjunct faculty because they often teach a large number of students (Avery, 2013). New instructors may not be familiar with the teaching roles librarians play. Even in the first three semesters of this collaboration, librarians at USD often found themselves working with new instructors or discovering that adjuncts who taught the class one semester were not scheduled to teach it the next. Without a specific directive to incorporate IL instruction into FYW classes, librarians had to continually cultivate relationships with writing instructors. The value of this engagement, of course, was that the library was collaborating with more faculty as it was making gains in reaching students. The next challenge to tackle was considering how best to assess the IL skills taught in FYW.

Other than interacting with them in class and being present while they conducted searches and asked questions, librarians had little way of knowing how much FYW students were retaining in the way of IL skills beyond informal reports of improved assignments from their instructors. Students' acquisition of IL skills has been assessed in a variety of ways in higher education, from pre-/post-tests to surveys or focus groups of faculty to measure their "perceptions of success" (White-Farnham & Gardner, 2014, p. 282). Since the initial focus of the library's collaboration with FYW was on building the program and reaching students, librarians did not have the opportunity to devise an assessment tool. Although there was interest from some instructors in a pre-/post-test, creating, testing, and implementing it would require further time and planning. Because IL is assessed at the university level for accreditation purposes, there was an intentional decision, if only temporary, to postpone assessment of IL in FYW so as not to duplicate efforts. Nevertheless, librarians did serve alongside discipline faculty as scorers of student work for university assessment in both CTIL and Writing. The chance to serve in this capacity created yet another opportunity for librarians to engage faculty and administrators in conversations about IL. Serving on university committees was the other opportunity for participating in meaningful discussion about the core curriculum and the role the library might play as IL programming evolves.

Librarians and university service

Librarians from Copley Library have been full members of the faculty for over 40 years and participate in faculty governance. Silva et al. (2017) note that faculty status can help to elevate the stature of librarians on campus as opposed to being staff members. Any further elevation of status for librarians at USD may be because of increased exposure through university committees. Johnson-Grau et al. (2016) note the crucial role of participating in faculty governance, especially in curriculum committees, to the success of their efforts in influencing conversations about IL. Similarly, librarians at USD sought to leverage their academic status to play a larger role in curriculum development. Serendipitously, university conversations about the appropriate place for CTIL began not long after the library initiated its partnership with FYW.

Following the Fall 2017 university assessment of student attainment of CTIL skills through the aforementioned Historical Inquiry classes, there was a growing interest in investigating a new home for this core competency. After the first full year of the core's implementation, faculty had a better understanding of what aspects were working well and what needed improvement. For CTIL, the question was whether learning outcomes of these competencies might be more effectively realized in another course or courses. Challenges of the present model included the heavy burden placed on faculty teaching Historical Inquiry courses and the large number of lower division courses with the CTIL competency, meaning CTIL was not formally embedded at the upper division level. At the beginning of the 2019 Spring semester, these conversations made their way to the university Core Curriculum Committee (CCC). As previously mentioned, there was already one librarian on this committee. The incoming library committee member was the Coordinator of Instruction. This meant that not only did the library have a potential role to play in shaping the curriculum, but it also had faculty working on the CCC with direct experience coordinating a successful project to embed IL sessions into core courses. Faculty outside of the Writing Program also knew about the partnership between FYW and the library and recognized the librarians involved with the CCC as being active in other IL initiatives at the university. When a CTIL Task Force was formed to investigate alternatives to embedding the CTIL competencies in Historical Inquiry courses, the librarians were asked to join. The Coordinator of Instruction was named as committee chair.

The CTIL Task Force's charge is to study the pros and cons of several different models of incorporating the competency into the core curriculum, such as flagging critical thinking and information literacy separately in courses across the curriculum or adding IL to FYW courses. The latter option would fit with the library/FYW partnership, but it would still mean IL would happen officially only at the lower division level. Librarians needed to be mindful of balancing their own goal of reaching a maximum number of first-year students with the curricular concern of placing IL in a way that would scaffold it across the curriculum and lend itself to assessing student attainment for core competencies.

The CTIL Task Force is undertaking its charge as of this chapter's writing. It will be required to discuss its findings at open faculty forums and department meetings and solicit feedback. The next step will be to present the research along with faculty feedback to the CCC, which will then make a recommendation for a new CTIL model in the core to the faculty of each unit granting undergraduate degrees. Challenges will inevitably arise, but being part of the process of curricular change is worth any setbacks. In two years, librarians proved that they could successfully engage faculty and were now an active part of the push to enhance student learning at USD.

Lessons learned

Seek more faculty input

In the push to reach as many students as possible through a first-year requirement, librarians initially did not spend enough time considering the concerns outside IL that could mean library instruction not always rating as a priority for those leading sections of FYW. Although they had multiple one-on-one conversations with the Writing Program Director and FYW faculty in addition to the meetings where the library collaboration was proposed, instruction sessions could have been more effective had there been an effort to seek faculty input by way of surveys or focus groups. As librarians learned with the charge of the CTIL task force, being supportive of faculty requires soliciting feedback to determine best practices on campus.

Question assumptions

Even though FYW does present an attractive option for IL instruction, the writing course is predominantly grounded in writing practice and rhetorical strategies. The two SLOs mentioned in this chapter speak to IL skills, but there is no research requirement *per se*. Other than simply not having the time to devote a class session to library instruction, the most common reason given by faculty for not collaborating with a librarian was that students analyzed writing and incorporated evidence into their assignments using course readings as opposed to outside sources. While recent successes suggest the library will continue to reach a large number of first year students through FYW, this may not be the only way to incorporate IL into the curriculum.

Build in assessment

Working with other faculty in sessions scoring both CTIL and Writing was illuminating for librarians working on the FYW partnership, chiefly for the conversations the sessions sparked with faculty about student attainment in addition to the value of seeing student work firsthand. Still, librarians have yet to incorporate formal assessment into the FYW library instruction sessions. Even if the IL core competency is not ultimately placed in FYW, there will still need to be assessment of student learning given the effort that goes in to reaching this many students. Assessments via online modules or pre-/post-tests are near the top of the priority list for program development.

Conclusion

To begin with the goal of starting a program that would impact student learning in the first year and end with participating in curriculum reform is more than the librarians could have hoped for. At the outset, they researched best IL instruction practices. This review proved doubly useful when they began serving on the CTIL Task Force and needed to research institutional practices for embedding these competencies into the curriculum. From an outreach standpoint, gains were made in reaching faculty and building relationships. Although the outcomes of these efforts are to be determined, the librarians are satisfied with progress so far and gratified by the response rate from FYW instructors requesting IL sessions and the overall improvement in library instruction. As they move to the next step of assessment, they can hopefully gain more insight into the efficacy of the instruction and, as will undoubtedly be necessary, further improve upon and augment the program to include undergraduate students at the lower and upper division levels.

References

American Library Association. (2015). *Framework for information literacy for higher education.* Retrieved from http://www.ala.org/acrl/standards/ilframework

Avery, S. (2013). Adjunct faculty and the library: A challenge for change. *College & Undergraduate Libraries, 20*(1), 25–39. doi:10.1080/10691316.2013.761049

Bowles-Terry, M. (2012). Library instruction and academic success: A mixed-methods assessment of a library instruction program. *Evidence Based Library and Information Practice, 7*(1), 82–95. doi:10.18438/B8PS4D

Buchanan, H. E., & McDonough, B. A. (2017). *The one-shot library instruction survival guide* (2nd ed.). Chicago, IL: American Library Association.

Dhawan, A., & Chen, C. J. (2014). Library instruction for first-year students. *Reference Services Review, 42*(3), 414–432. doi:10.1108/RSR-04-2014-0006

Goldman, C., Turnbow, D., Roth, A., & Friedman, L. (2016). Creating an engaging library orientation: First year experience courses at University of California, San Diego. *Communications in Information Literacy, 10*(1), 81–98. doi:10/.15760/comminfolit.2016.10.1.16

Johnson-Grau, G., Archambault, S.G., Acosta, E.S., & McLean, L. (2016). Patience, persistence, and process: Embedding a campus-wide information literacy program across the curriculum. *Journal of Academic Librarianship, 42*(6), 750–756. doi:10.1016/j.acalib.2016.10.013

Morphew, C., Ward, K., & Wolf-Wendel, L. (2017). Contingent faculty composition and utilization: Perspectives from independent colleges and universities. *New Directions for Institutional Research, 176*, 67–81. doi:10.1002/ir.20245

Riehle, C. F., & Weiner, S. A. (2013). High-impact educational practices: An exploration of the role of information literacy. *College & Undergraduate Libraries, 20*(2), 127–142. doi:10.1080/10691316.2013.789658

Silva, E., Galbraith, Q., & Groesbeck, M. (2017). Academic librarians' changing perceptions of faculty status and tenure. *College & Research Libraries, 78*(4), 428–441. doi:10.5860/crl.78.4.428

University of San Diego. (2017). *University of San Diego Core Curriculum Fall 2017.* Retrieved from https://www.sandiego.edu/curriculum/documents/core-curriculum.pdf

WASC Senior College and University Commission. (2013). *2013 handbook of accreditation revised.* Retrieved from https://www.wscuc.org/book/export/html/924

White-Farnham, J., & Gardner, C. C. (2014). Crowdsourcing the curriculum: Information literacy instruction in first-year writing. *Reference Services Review, 42*(2), 277–292. doi:10.1108/RSR-09-2013-0046

8

FISCAL FITNESS THROUGH FINANCIAL LITERACY

Rosalind K. Lett

Bringing fiscal fitness to a community through financial literacy takes strategic community-focused planning, teamwork, and a real passion to empower your community. Financial literacy can positively influence a community and help citizens to build capacity and learn techniques to manage debt. Writing a FINRA (Financial Industry Regulatory Authority) Smart Investing at Your Library Grant proposal for $100,000 was the catalyst that enabled us to start a comprehensive financial initiative in Clayton County, Georgia, USA. After examining demographic information from the 2010 census, we were able to identify target audiences with the greatest needs in the cities in Clayton County, Georgia (Jonesboro, Riverdale, Morrow, Lake City, Forest Park, College Park, Rex, Lovejoy, and Ellenwood). To identify specific needs unique to the Clayton County Community, research was conducted. This research identified citizens who are financially disenfranchised, unbanked, and un-bankable, meaning they do not have bank accounts and have very limited financial resources in the county. Keeping this in mind, we set out to create smart goals, objectives, and outcomes to provide fiscal fitness for all members of our community.

The Clayton County Library System serves 285,153 (Census.gov, 2017) citizens in a county that is home to the Hartsfield-Jackson International Airport, the world's busiest airport in Atlanta, GA. Yet, although the airport generates hundreds of millions of dollars in revenue, the impact on Clayton County citizens is nominal. The average median household income in 2017 was $42,470 (Census.gov, 2017) up from 2014 when the median income was $39,699.

The Clayton County Library System (CCLS) serves a diverse population consisting of African Americans, Caucasians, Hispanics, Vietnamese, Asians, and others, with a staff of approximately 95 employees, located in six library branches (a headquarters and five branches). The library staff have extensive experience coordinating long-running, cohesive, and well-attended programs, such as our summer reading program, entrepreneurial training, and workshops which were highly valued in the community.

The Clayton County Library System utilized a FINRA grant to offer financial literacy training through programs, simulations and resources to targeted demographics within the community. Our project called "Healthy, Wealthy and Wise" focused on four specific targeted demographic groups: entrepreneurs, financially disenfranchised families, seniors, and youth. We chose these four target groups to help augment their opportunities for lifelong learning, and enhance their chances for self-sufficiency through financial literacy training. Our program provides the fundamentals for individual prosperity and economic independence to survive, and connect them to resources within the county that help improve their quality of life. Demographics show that school graduation rates are low in Clayton County with 32% of the population graduating high school and 13% with college degrees. Only 51% of residents own property in Clayton County, so there was plenty of opportunity to work with citizens on Home Ownership (United Way Atlanta, n.d.). Surveys of citizen visiting the library, seniors at the senior centers, entrepreneurs at the library hot topic sessions, and youth at youth programming provided data to help us determine which populations to target.

We chose to approach schools offering "Banking on our Future" because the schools have five financial literacy modules that must be incorporated into the school curriculum and our program satisfied these requirements. credit and money management along with home ownership were identified needs for Clayton County Families. Reality Check was offered for our teens to stimulate understanding financial realities, Money Smart activities like make and take piggy bank crafts for early learners and fraud and money management, estate planning, and investing for our seniors.

Goals

The goals for our project were divided to fit each unique demographic group, the entrepreneurs, senior citizens, youth, and disenfranchised families. The goal for the entrepreneurs was to increase their capacity to become knowledgeable about business creation, financing, and key issues effecting business management.

Based on the data from the United Way data (United Way Atlanta, n.d.), we realized that financially disenfranchised families and their children were more likely not to have the skills that they need to manage money and credit. The limited capability of our low-income citizens to increase or leverage their funds and the growing gap between access to finance and financial capability were criteria used to select this group. Thus, we felt that our financially disenfranchised families would be better equipped to manage their finances after attending our programs including sessions on budgeting, credit and money management, and fiscal responsibility. Our goal for the youth was for them to become more familiar with the language of money, to learn to write a check, to be able to develop a budget and to manage their money more effectively (savings and spending). The goal for seniors was to increase knowledge and interest in and utilization of library offerings.

A goal was also established for the library and its staff. Library staff was expected to gain greater competency in handling finance-related reference questions and increased confidence in their ability to answer finance-related reference questions. To support this goal, staff was trained at a staff development day workshop to work with children and families. Staff reviewed available financial resources and handouts that we were making available to the public. As a result of the project, the library was expected to improve its visibility among entrepreneurs, seniors, and citizens seeking personal financial information.

The information about our programs was marketed on our website, through email blast on the county email system, flyers posted in our branch libraries and in many locations around the community. We also used social media (Facebook, Twitter, Snap Chat, and other social media platforms), sent out text messages, posted events on EventBrite, and we used word-of-mouth marketing at outreach events.

How the project started

Our program started in 2015 after receiving notification that we'd been awarded $100,000 for our Financial Literacy Grant. We began with training for the Principle Investigator and Grant Coordinator at a Federal Industry Regulatory Authority (FINRA) workshop held in Chicago, Illinois at the Midwinter Conference of the American Library Association (ALA). After attending the workshop and training in Chicago, our in-house work began with the formation of the working groups for each target audience. Four teams of five staff members each were formed, with each team being headed by an assistant director. These teams were comprised of staff who volunteered or who worked with the target population. Once the teams were formed they reviewed the grant focus to customize training, adapt workshops, select simulations, and identify ways to connect with their target audience. Teams were excited about planning and learning about financial literacy and how we would work to change the financial literacy proficiency levels of the community.

Youth

Prior to us introducing our program and visiting schools, we formed a partnership with Operation Hope. Operation Hope is a global agency focused on financial literacy and empowerment. This partnership was facilitated by our library board chairperson, who felt that our program was a match to the mission of Operation Hope. Operation Hope introduced us to their curriculum, the participant and teacher's guides they used to provide instruction. They allowed us to use their curriculum "Banking on our Future" with the third, fifth, and eighth-grade students. This curriculum was easy to present and easy for the students to comprehend. They provided workbooks, calculators, and incentives for us to give to the classes.

To gain school system buy-in we obtained the Clayton County School Media Specialist and Coordinators list. Library staff met with the specialist to discuss project goals and explain benefits for students and teachers. We shared our project approach as a win-win opportunity, that consisted of onsite visits to the school's third-, fifth-, and eighth-grade classrooms. The students were taught the language of money, how to budget, how to save money, and how to spend their money more effectively. We would use library staff volunteers but also volunteers from the corporate partners of Operations Hope.

Overcoming barriers and moving forward

Although we had gotten support from administration when we wrote the grant, we encountered significant challenges. Scheduling training sessions became an issue, due to conflicts with testing, teacher being unsure and unwilling to commit to the training and no clear support coming from school administration. With support from the top being so critical, we re-strategize our buy-in approach. A personal connection was made with a school board member who introduced us to an assistant superintendent who understood the value of financial literacy for the students. We met face-to-face to present our case for introducing financial literacy and illustrating the instruction time our program would save the teachers. The assistant principal allowed us to present at a meeting of principals, teachers, and media specialist. The message that resonated with the teachers and media specialist was the fulfillment of five of their financial literacy teaching module requirements. Alas, the return-on-investment was realized and the fact that the teachers would regain some of their time because we would be conducting the training. Principals and teachers began immediately contacting us to schedule sessions for their students. The request started coming in faster than we could get them scheduled. This resulted in a world-wind school tour where we scheduled several schools over a four-week period to get them in before the end of the school year.

We planned to offer some of our youth programming in-house at our libraries and at the Clayton County parks and recreation Centers. Our youth services team members integrated engaging money lessons, hands-on programs, and county-wide story times into our summer reading program and Money Smart Week.

For the sixth grade, and older children we hosted extension service simulations to teach the day-to-day realities of life, living with a shortage of money and the associated stressors, using a program called Reality Checks. We initially worked through the parks and recreation and library branches to recruit participants, like our home school groups. We found it more effective to collaborate with local children's agencies, identified teen groups and to collaborate with organized groups like Girl Scouts. These participants were engaged in interactive learning lessons and a variety of money-based activities during Money Smart Week in April of each year.

We planned to use resources, such as Love your Money, Money Smart for Young Adults, and Generation Money, to design our series of biweekly inter-active teen sessions. We changed our plans after the extension service allowed us to participate in Reality Check, to experience firsthand what the kids would experience. We realized how quickly and easily we could set up the poverty simulation, and how much the kids enjoyed the experience. This discovery led us to use the simulation, which only lasts for one hour. Each 15 minutes being equivalent to a week. Participants were given life scenario, with jobs, salary, and family dynamics. Kids purchased housing, transportation, child care, food, and all of the needs and wants of life, living within their means for a month. The challenges of daily survival became crystal clear after the first 15 minutes, when students began to purchase necessities and realize that their money was not going to last the entire month. The students began to strategize about how to survive the month. Many students got part-time jobs, while others shared living arrangements and modes of transportation to save money. When the sim-ulation ended, the teens talked about the expense of childcare and the things that surprised them about living through a month paying bills and surviving on a fixed income.

Our FINRA Grant funding lasted two years. Since that time, other commu-nity partners were solicited who support the program as it continues to offer fi-nancial literacy to the school system. We are transforming our program using an interactive digital-based software program called Everfi. Everfi is designed with modules for elementary, middle School, and high school students, so that kids from all schools, in all grades have access to financial literacy training, through self-paced instruction modules. We are launching Everfi through the library so that the home school kids and kids from charter schools as well as the Clayton County school system will have access to the modules.

Entrepreneurs: business finance and beginning investing

For the entrepreneurs program, our Instructors provided financial literacy train-ing based on the Financial Industry Regulatory Authority (FINRA) resources and the Small Business Association (SBA) resources conducting interactive class-room and flipped classroom style workshops. We worked with the Economic Development Department, Small Business Development Center (SBDC), and country human resources, to offer "Eggs and Issues" an early morning version of "Lunch and Learn", to reach entrepreneurs and county employees interested in starting a business. After experimenting with daytime and evening sessions, we realized based on participant feedback and attendance, that the most suc-cessful sessions for entrepreneurs were held on Thursday nights. We created an eight-week multi-session evening workshop series offered at our headquarters and Riverdale branch. We offered business development training and resources to educate county residents in starting a business. We supplemented this training with special financial topic workshops, boot camps, offsite business expos, databases, and web resource training. These resources were available to the public, county departments, and community partners.

While our original plan was to create a series of workshops, the financial literacy curriculum for entrepreneurs used by Operation Hope was shared with us. We used their curriculum template as a guide and created our eight-week session curriculum. Our sessions' topics included: How to Start a Business, Selecting a Business Structure, Conducting Market Research, Risk Management for Business, and more. We conducted the eight-week workshop series for four weeks with a one-week break, followed by the second four weeks. Based on feedback from the entrepreneur's weekly surveys and participant feedback sessions conducted during our off week, we re-aligned our class sessions using the Small Business Administration (SBA) training modules to include more in-depth training options. We did this because the instructors indicated that the modules were easier for them to teach from, and the participants shared that they needed resources that were easier to understand when they reviewed them at home after the sessions. These modules offered template PowerPoints, Participant and instructor's guides, and follow-up resources. The participants requested resources that they could refer back to after the sessions were over. Many of the SBA programs are online and have supporting articles or useful resources linked from the site. We also included more experienced entrepreneurs to share their stories, and their mistakes to provide the entrepreneurs with a vivid picture of business ownership. An extra element that we included when we began the series after the funding had ended was to engage entrepreneurs who could provide the participants with a tangible take away. We had sessions on preparing a business plan, a vision board, grant writing, and other skill sets that would benefit all entrepreneurs. We also provided sessions for small business owners and entrepreneurs on financial management, financial accounting tools, raising capital, market research, web-based business resources and making Investment decisions using web-based business information resources such as *Mergent, A to Z,* and *Career Accelerator* databases.

Disenfranchised families: personal finance and decision making

We worked through organizations that serve financially disenfranchised families such as Habitat for Humanities, the Department of Families and Children's Services (DFACS), Kinship Care, the Clayton County Health Dept. and other organizations to identify target families who needed financial literacy training. Using instructors from the Clayton County Cooperative Extension Service, and local community service agencies, we presented financial strategies for financial planning, banking, budgeting, saving, managing credit, and other personal money management topics. We incorporated resources such as Financial Planning Opportunities for People of all Incomes, English and Spanish Personal Finance e-guides and other FINRA resources to address these topics. Our intent was to offer some of these sessions at faith-based organizations in the community. Local churches have a history of collaborating with the library. We found the library to be more conducive to our training due to computer equipment and internet access needs but we heavily recruited in local churches. The majority of our sessions were held at our headquarters and branch libraries. Programs included a combination of lectures and hands-on computer-based training using laptops or digital devices at offsite community locations.

We provided handouts outlining key components, website links pointing to FINRA's financial literacy training, library guides with access instructions and other useful financial literacy information. Participants received day planners for bill pay schedule planning, calculators to compute payments and interest, flash drives to save pertinent financial information, library bags to transport their resources and other swag (pens, markers, pencils, etc.). At the sessions, tips for using these tools and others were shared. After completion of a few eight-week entrepreneurial series, we engaged a videographer to film the entrepreneurial sessions.

The financially disenfranchised members of our community were categorized in several ways. This diverse group included immigrants (with problems understanding our currency system), and predatory lending targets (people victimized by pay day and title loan vendors). New residents of Georgia (the hardest state to get a bank account in), and other non-banked groups (college students trying to get checking accounts and people with bad credit) were also included. Georgia ranks fifth in the nation in the "unbanked" (people who don't have bank accounts and use cash or alternatives to bankcards, i.e. fee-based debit cards). Unbanked are described by the Federal Depository Insurance Corporation (FDIC) as adults without an account at a bank or financial institution. Our approach through faith-based organizations was successful in identifying participants and providing library community engagement opportunities. However, we recognized that integrating our program into churches such as the Vietnamese church we would need to identify ambassadors to help us gain the trust of these community groups and translate our materials into other languages.

Seniors: retirement, financial disaster planning, and estate planning

We worked closely with Clayton County Senior Services department. This organization has over 10,000 members who visit four senior centers around the county. Two of the most popular centers average 200–300 senior member visits per day. We surveyed the seniors in the centers to determine what programs they wanted. The seniors requested classes on financial strategies that included basic investing; estate planning; retirement preparation; financial disaster planning and savings. We included Consumer Financial Protection Bureau (CFPB) and FINRA resources on savings and money management, particularly the Retirement and Savings calculators, and the Making Ends Meet toolkit.

We visited the senior centers offering Habitat for Humanity's sessions on home repairs. Their program required participants to take financial literacy classes. We also participated in Mayfest (the annual senior event filled with educational opportunities, entertainment, games and fun) sponsored by the senior center. At Mayfest we manned a table with financial information, games and incentives branded with the library financial literacy "Healthy, Wealthy and Wise" logo.

Team and teaching

We used a team approach to addressing the needs of each of our groups. We created working groups comprised of a team leader, a community liaison and 4–5 team members for each target group. We found out that having a community-focused, philanthropic-minded coordinator helped us streamline the process and keep our teams and project on track. We used the flipped classroom approach to train-the-trainer workshops for our team leaders, library staff, and instructors. This approach entails providing handouts and readings ahead of the class session so that informed discussion and question and answers can be covered in an interactive class.

Outcomes

Entrepreneurs

Based on the results of our surveys and continuous participant feedback, we concluded that 65% of our participants had a better understanding funding a business and options available to help them save and leverage their money. Many of these entrepreneurs became regular participants in our continuing entrepreneurial training and come to the library frequently to use library resources. As a result of this training, some have written or re-written business plans, and others have changed their business structure. Many of the participants have launched their businesses and come in the library regularly to use resources (such as *Mergent*, *A to Z,* and other web-based business sites) to support their market research and business management efforts.

Financially disenfranchised families

The participants expressed satisfaction with the information that they received in the credit and money management sessions. This information included how to use credit cards wisely to increase their credit scores and how to find budget worksheets online to develop a budget. When the instructors offered one-on-one follow-up sessions with the class participants to review their credit history and dispute errors, 77% of participants set up individual appointments with the instructor on the day of the session. Several of the participants improved their credit scores enough to purchase homes.

Seniors

Senior program participants expressed on surveys, feeling more comfortable dealing with debt, credit, and saving, and they now are familiar with locating financial resources. Seniors understand the steps needed to prevent themselves from being victims of fraud or identity theft. Their comprehension extends to managing money with a budget, investing their money, and protecting finances during natural disasters.

Youth

During the workshops at the Clayton County schools a "thumbs up, thumbs down" assessment was used. The majority of the students (classes averaged 30 students) 90–95% indicated that they understood what financial dignity was and could give us an example of someone who was leading a dignified life. They understood the basics of budgeting after participating in the build a budget for a summer vacation exercise. The students were excited to learn to write a check and explore financial topics like debit cards and identity theft.

Challenges and lessons learned

Entrepreneurs

We learned the value of participant attendance at each series session to retain knowledge and prioritize their business processes. We learned not to assume that seasoned business people follow proven techniques for business set up. Many entrepreneurs didn't know how to conduct market research, choose a business structure, market their business, not to mention how to brand their business on social media. We discovered it's more cost effective to use the Federal Depository Insurance Corp (FDIC), Consumer Financial Protection Bureau (CFPB), Small Business Administration (SBA), and Financial Industry Regulatory Authority (FINRA) resources with evaluation instruments built in, for online and onsite surveys.

Financially disenfranchised families

We discovered increasing advertising in schools and at community meetings, in many formats, resulted in increased participation. Dispelling the assumption that everyone has internet access, or that all people seek information from the Internet, was important to remember when advertising.

We realized a need to translate handouts, presentations and library materials into other languages. We realized locating facilitators who can present in Spanish or Vietnamese was not an easy task but needed in our community.

Youth

We learned how helpful it is to incorporate planning sessions with the teachers to provide a project overview. We found that conducting a teacher train-the-trainer session at least a week prior to the workshops was extremely valuable. We discovered that creating a template, so that every volunteer instructor was teaching the same lessons using the same examples, was more effective (e.g. Summer Vacation Budget Plan).

After some trial and error, we learned that offering classes 2–3 days a week in school clusters worked better with staff and volunteer schedules. We found that we needed to recruit more community volunteers to teach, thus reducing staff overwork, and burnout.

Seniors

With the seniors we discovered timing is everything. We reconsidered offering programs during the lunch break, changing to before or after lunch, because seniors want to socialize during lunch. We got better participation when attending seniors supported activities, such as MayFest and other community events targeted to seniors. Seniors love giveaways, handouts, and incentives. We gave pens, lunch bags, playing cards, and tote bags as giveaways. We made giveaways available at all sessions and made them available in the senior centres when we conducted surveys.

Overall

It's more cost effective to purchase flash drives and put all handouts on the drives. Make sure the person chosen as the outreach coordinator is an energetic, extroverted person with experience making community connections. Making sure our partners understood their roles and were willing to fulfill those roles was also important. We always provided snacks and water so participants would have something to eat.

Recommendations

Start with a working group and get them engaged early. Have the group conduct peer training. Recruit volunteers early so they can experience the entire process. Plan events at least 60 days in advance so that they can be well advertised through multiple media channels. Do not forget about the technically challenged. Have print and non-print session notices available. Advertise in places where people congregate (i.e. grocery stores, churches, schools, sporting events, and non-profit agencies).

Start your project off with a solid coordinator who has outreach and partnership building expertise. Be willing to change coordinators early if planning is done but deliverables are not completed.

Remind speakers to come prepared in case the Internet is down, with handouts, props, and a good grasp of the subject matter. Talk about your program to identify new presenters and partners. Be open to finding support, sometimes from unlikely partners.

Part five: evaluation plan

We hired an evaluator with many years of experience writing and evaluating library grants using the Objective-Based Evaluation Method (OBE). Due to an unforeseen illness we had to find a replacement evaluator who relocated to Washington D.C. in the middle of our project. Therefore, she didn't experience as much of the project firsthand as planned. However, using strategically planned site visits, email, text, Skype, and other social media helped us get materials transported quickly, surveys tallied, and our OBE completed on time and within budget.

The evaluator worked closely with us to develop the surveys. We used a professional survey package called CVENT to customize our surveys, gather real-time responses, compile the data and report the results. The workshop instructors and program coordinator distributed anonymous surveys at each session. Evaluation data was a rolling process as well as a cumulative one, which allowed us to immediately adjust our programming according to the feedback we received.

a   **Entrepreneurs:** Our most involved evaluation was for this demographic. In the business introduction, multi-session workshop evaluations were reviewed immediately following classes to enable us to reach out and offer additional resources when needed. Pre and post evaluations were used to track financial literacy building behavior, including: how comfortable participants felt choosing a structure for their business, researching companies, targeting markets, and using web-based research tools and library resources. We used program improvement surveys to gauge our efficacy, and refine our program and format as requested by the participants.

Workshop instructors received the compiled results of the pre and post evaluations along with the professional evaluator (who had no names or other identifiers). Surveys administered onsite for optimal participation proved successful, which was contrary to our initial plan, where we planned to allow participants to complete surveys days after the sessions.

b   **Financially Disenfranchised:** The "credit and money management" session not only had surveys but also offered the opportunity for one-on-one counseling sessions. We used pre and post evaluations to track personal financial management behavior, including financial planning and management improvements (such as meeting savings goals or improving credit scores), and evidence of participants making better financial decisions.

Programming partners

It is important to acknowledge the project partners who collaborated on this effort. The Clayton Collaborative Authority (CCA) is one of our community partners that administered the funds.

Operation Hope provided us with curriculum and facilitators for onsite school sessions and introduced us to community volunteers who helped us at the schools. They also conducted train-the-trainer sessions for library staff.

The extension service provided instructors and the resources for the reality check. Habitat for Humanity provided participants for our financial literacy class

TABLE 8.1 Programming partners: each programming partner had their own outreach channels

Partners	Role
Clayton County Collaborative	501 c3 financial pass-through wrote checks, and held funds
Clayton County Parks & Recreation Dept.	Promoted workshops and recruited participants
Clayton County Senior Services	Promoted workshops and recruited participants Provides space for training sessions
Clayton County Commissioners	Provided advertising and participants
Kinship Care	Provided participants both grandparents and grandchildren
Clayton County Habitat for Humanities	Recruited participants and directed them to our financial literacy sessions
Girl Scouts of America NW Council	Participated in financial literacy sessions and earned badges
Operation Hope	Workshop facilitators, curriculum for schools, volunteers, credit and money management classes, homeownership
Clayton County Extension Service	Facilitated teen reality check
Clayton County Chamber of Commerce	Advertised, referred participants, trainers
Clayton County Economic Development	Workshop facilitators
Clayton County School System	Provided participants in 3rd, 5th, and 8th grade to participate in Banking on our future
Clayton State University	Workshop participants, advertising, provides space for training sessions
Clayton County Community Services	Information on county licenses and permits
Clayton County Government	Advertising, participant for training sessions
Local Business Owners	Participants in training sessions, sharing experiences
Clayton County Non-Profits	Provides space for training sessions

who needed training to qualify for their home repair program. They also hosted training sessions that we facilitated.

Senior services provided sites for our senior training, helped advertise sessions, and provided participants for senior sessions. The Clayton County Commissioners (CCC) allowed us to advertise in their newsletters that were distributed throughout their county via the website.

Kinship Care was a source of senior participants and children to participate in the programs and interactive activities offered to increase financial literacy. Girl Scouts provided access to local Girl Scout troops to participate in financial literacy arts and crafts and to work on financial literacy badges (Table 8.1).

Other outcomes

The library ordered financial literacy books, videos, games, and other materials to support our financial literacy programs. Each branch library displays their financial literacy books and report significant use by the public. We added a texting service to our marketing efforts to push notices to our participants and worked with a marketing company to help us advertise through our newsletter, on radio, and through advertising videos. We were asked to participate in a debt management workshop at Clayton State University sponsored by the Leadership Clayton Class of 2018.

The aftermath

The grant funding has ended but our program is still alive and growing and our entrepreneurs and SBA programs are ongoing through established collaborations. We have concurrently offered our SBA training for entrepreneurs at the Riverdale branch. We offer BB&T Bank's Home Buyers Program and some of their Entrepreneur's Workshop. SunTrust Bank supported our 11-week Entrepreneurs Session in partnership with Operation Hope. We are also continuing to offer Operation Hope's Credit and Money Management for Small Business and Entrepreneurs.

We are introducing Everfi to the students through the library. While they are contemplating how to introduce this software, the library is taking the lead. Links are being set up on our website, and lessons for home schoolers and other youth are being piloted. We participate annually in Money Smart Week and the county-wide Financial Literacy Read-Aloud. We engage the students with make and take money crafts, boot camps, and other interactive competency building activities.

For disenfranchised families, we continue to conduct "credit and money management classes" and home ownership classes facilitated by operation hope. Participants are still able to get individual credit counseling and "down payment assistance" for buying a house.

We continue to offer workshops to seniors on fraud, identity theft, estate planning, saving, and investing. We participate in other senior programs as well as the annual Mayfest celebration. In 2019, we rolled out a four-topic workshop series for seniors on Scams and Fraud Protection, Identity Theft, Financial Care Givers, and Basic Emailing in partnership with BB&T Bank.

New audiences

We have collaborated with the Clayton County Veteran's Advisory Board to offer financial literacy programs to veterans. Clayton County has over 24,000 veterans, many of whom need as much help as other citizens in managing money and credit. Lastly, the library is collaborating with emergency medical services to introduce them to the financial disaster preparedness resources for them to share with the community.

Our goals with "Healthy, Wealthy and Wise" were to change the way people in Clayton County manage, save, invest, and learn about financial literacy. We endeavored to increase their knowledge base and increase the participants' capacity to make informed financial decisions; earn wisely, spend, share and save money, manage their money effectively; and understand the basic concepts and skills needed for personal fiscal fitness. This was accomplished through training, community outreach, and collaborating with our county resources and community partners.

Financial literacy is a permanent part of our Clayton County Library System services, and we will continue to offer classes, programs, interactive simulations, book collections, kids financial make and take crafts, county-wide story time, games, financial disaster preparedness, credit and money management sessions, avoiding identity theft, and many more exciting and engaging financial literacy programs. In Clayton County we continue to invest our time and efforts to make our citizens "Healthy, Wealthy and Wise".

References

Census.gov. (2017). *U.S. Census Bureau QuickFacts: Clayton County, Georgia*. Retrieved from http://www.census.gov/quickfacts/fact/table/claytoncountygeorgia
United Way Atlanta. (n.d.). Child-well-being-overview. Retrieved from http://www.unitedwayatlanta.org/child-well-being-overview

9

EXPANDING HEALTH INFORMATION OUTREACH THROUGH ACADEMIC HEALTH SCIENCE PARTNERS

Elizabeth Kiscaden and Jacqueline Leskovec

Introduction

The National Network of Libraries of Medicine (NNLM) is a program of the U.S. National Library of Medicine (NLM), carried out through eight Regional Medical Libraries (RMLs) and a national network of over 6,800 members (National Network of Libraries of Medicine, 2018). NNLM was established through the Medical Library Assistance Act of 1965 and was originally known as the Regional Medical Library Program (RMLP). The Program was designed to improve medical school libraries in the United States and their ability to provide access to biomedical information (Bunting, 1987). In the 1980s and 1990s, the mission of NNLM expanded to include a focus on health information outreach to the public. NLM and the RMLs developed consumer health information resources to support the public's need for health information at an appropriate reading level. This expansion resulted in the development of the current mission statement and the name of the program, the National Network of Libraries of Medicine:

> The mission of NNLM is to advance the progress of medicine and improve public health by providing all U.S. health professionals with equal access to biomedical information and improving the public's access to information to enable them to make informed decisions about their health.
>
> *(National Network of Libraries of Medicine, 2018)*

Each of the eight RMLs is academic health sciences libraries funded under a competitive, renewable five-year grant awarded by NLM. The Regions include the Middle Atlantic (MAR), Southeastern / Atlantic (SEA), Greater Midwest (GMR), MidContinental (MCR), New England (NER), Pacific Southwest

(PSR), South Central (SCR), and the Pacific Northwest (PNR). These eight RMLs conduct outreach, including funding health information projects, and training on NLM resources within their respective Region.

In particular, the consumer health information resources that NNLM promotes and provides training on are those freely available resources created and maintained by NLM, including popular online databases such as PubMed® and MedlinePlus®. PubMed is a bibliographic database of biomedical literature which contains nearly 30 million citations, pulling primarily from MEDLINE®, an authoritative index maintained by NLM. MedlinePlus, designed specifically for the health consumer, contains information on over 1,000 health-related topics and aggregates content from trusted sources, such as the American Heart Association and Mayo Clinic, in addition to those of the National Institutes of Health and other U.S. government health-related databases.

The partnership presented here is the Partner Outreach Library (POL) Program implemented by the GMR during the 2016–2021 grant period. Hardin Library for the Health Sciences at the University of Iowa serves as the RML for the GMR. The office is located within Hardin Library and consists of a staff of six professional librarians and one full-time support staff, dedicated to serving the NNLM mission. The Region spans ten states along the upper Midwest, from the Dakotas east to Kentucky, and contains over 1,100 active institutional members.[1] The diversity of the Region ranges from major metropolitan cities (Chicago, Cincinnati, Columbus, and Cleveland) to rural, Appalachian, and tribal outpost organizations.

The partner outreach library program

The purpose of the Partner Outreach Library Program is to engage academic health sciences libraries within the Region to perform health information outreach on behalf of the GMR. Given the geographic size of the area, the vast number of institutional members (approximately one-sixth the entire Network), and the limited number of staff working within the GMR office, the Program relies upon partnerships with these health sciences libraries to extend its reach throughout the GMR's ten states.[2] These libraries are designated Partner Outreach Libraries (POL) and form a network that has an outreach mission to the state and the region. The program has served the GMR for nearly 20 years in one capacity or another and has been through a series of revisions throughout the various grant periods.

The Program, formerly called the Outreach Library Program, began during the 2001–2006 NLM funding period when the RML was located at the University of Illinois at Chicago Library of the Health Sciences. Following a similar program initiated by the NNLM South Central Region (SCR)[3], the Outreach Library Program was formed by a group of health sciences libraries who shared a mission of outreach. The GMR established a Memorandum of Understanding (MOU), which outlined the Program objectives and expectations, and each library was awarded the same amount, varying from $2,000 to $5,000 per year, depending upon the GMR budget. At the end of the year, libraries submitted final project reports, summarizing their efforts to meet the objectives listed in the MOU, and invoiced the GMR. During the 2016–2021 grant period, a change in the funding mechanism of the NNLM program meant it was no longer possible for the office to continue non-competitive stipends.

Unable to continue the Program as designed, the GMR drafted a proposal by which the outreach libraries operate under a pay-per-service model. Instead of annual stipends, libraries perform mutually agreed upon outreach activities, such as training or exhibiting, and submit invoices for the activities completed. The GMR then reimburses the libraries for costs involved in the activity, including transportation, printing, registration, lodging, personnel time, and other related costs. The redesigned Program, now known as the Partner Outreach Library (POL) Program, evolved over two years of process exchange and experimentation in partnership with the libraries and librarians in the group.

Under this new model, the network of Partner Outreach Libraries still had to complete an MOU with the GMR. Criteria for inclusion into the program are as follows:

- A mission of health information outreach to the community
- Qualified health information professionals with time dedicated to outreach activities
- Active membership in the NNLM
- Library staff familiarity with NLM/NIH resources

As outlined in the MOU, libraries will be reimbursed for activities undertaken on behalf of the GMR, will be funded to host up to two traveling exhibitions[4] from the National Library of Medicine (NLM) each year, and are invited to participate in quarterly online meetings coordinated by the GMR office. Quarterly meetings provide a platform not only by which the GMR can share information on NLM resources and NNLM initiatives, but the Partner Outreach Library can convey concerns, share successes, and inquire about potential outreach venues. The fact that the participating libraries and the GMR are considered partners has strengthened the Program. The feedback and ideas that the POLs provide during the quarterly meetings and at other times throughout the year assure that both the needs of the library and the GMR are met.

The Network Librarian within the GMR office coordinates and supports libraries in the Program. This staff member organizes activities, provides resources to participating libraries, and reports on the program to the office. Resources may include brochures, bookmarks, websites, or handouts requested by the POL or recommended by GMR staff for a given event. Libraries in the Program have access to an online guide which includes tools for activity reporting, invoicing, and shared curricula that may be used at other events. A newly designed POL digital badge is included in the guide (see Figure 9.1). POLs can

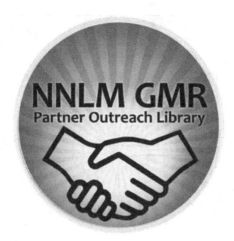

FIGURE 9.1   Partner Outreach Library digital badge.

use the badge on their library websites, display during outreach venues, and add to their email signatures to indicate participation in the Program. Also available in the guide is a Proposed Partner Outreach Activity Form used by participants to propose outreach activities in their communities.

The Network Librarian reviews submissions received through the form, responds to confirm that the event supports the NNLM mission, and may recommend resources and educational materials. Proposed activities are tracked via a spreadsheet provided by the survey tool. In this way, communication about activities is less likely to be lost in email. The spreadsheet is maintained as a way not only to track POL activities, but also to provide an easy way to report on POL outreach to GMR staff and NLM, and act as a way to follow through on invoicing.

The Partner Outreach Library Event flowchart (see Figure 9.2) maps out the process by which an outreach opportunity is identified and submitted to the GMR. The GMR reviews the activity, and if approved, notifies the POL and provides support materials such as handouts or other instructional materials as needed. Once the POL completes the activity, the appropriate evaluation form is completed online and an Activity Report (AR) is submitted. The Network Librarian reviews the form for completeness and once approved, provides a pdf copy of the AR for the POLs files. The final step in the process is invoicing and payment to the POL's institution.

One advantage of a network of outreach libraries is that these librarians are acquainted with the health information needs within their state. Local activities might include outreach to AIDs-affected communities, providing resources on rural health hazards, reaching out to seniors in need of digital access, eliminating food deserts, or providing first responders with tools to battle environmental disasters. Libraries in the Program have connections to local health and community

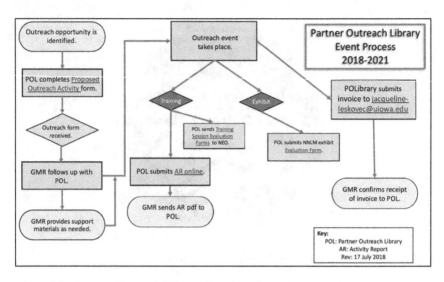

FIGURE 9.2   Partner Outreach Library flowchart for events.

organizations, such as hospitals, public libraries, schools, and senior centers, and can more easily form local connections. From a perspective of maximizing the limited budget of the GMR, local outreach librarians required less transportation, personnel time, and lodging costs than would be required to send GMR staff across the region.

While most outreach activities are submitted by the POLs via the Proposed Partner Outreach Activity Form, the GMR also solicits support from the POLs when a potential outreach activity is identified. POLs are asked to present and/or exhibit on behalf of the GMR at annual meetings for health professionals, educators, and librarians within their states. As an example, one POL in Ohio partnered with GMR staff to exhibit at the North American Hispanic Nurses conference held in Cleveland. These coordinated sessions provide an opportunity for both NNLM and the partnering library to showcase their resources and services, such as how to access multi-lingual and other free NLM resources, techniques for searching the professional literature through PubMed®, and ways of obtaining full-text articles.

Additionally, participating libraries may be included within large outreach projects funded by the GMR. For example, the office funded a project at an organization in Lakeville, Minnesota. As a component of this project, the POL in Minnesota provided the health information instruction component of the project. The librarian trained several classes of high-school students on how to locate reliable health information online, emphasizing NLM resources. Beyond funded projects, when the GMR receives a request for a presentation in a public library, community organization, or other venue, the office will contact the nearest POL and provide the library with the opportunity to provide the instruction on behalf of the office.

The Program is intentionally designed as a partnership, not only in the sense that it was co-developed with partner libraries, but in that the library participants and the GMR identify outreach opportunities. In this way the GMR office can share its expertise in outreach, NLM resources, and the NNLM mission; the POLs can contribute outreach opportunities meaningful to their constituents. POLs are enthusiastic about pursuing outreach opportunities, and the GMR works around schedules and staffing levels as needed. While participating institutions must be willing to perform outreach in the state, no participant has been removed from the program due to an inability to take on an opportunity presented by the office. The input of the POLs is essential to the success of the Program since it provides a sense of ownership between partners.

The Program has been successful in extending the reach of the GMR through a significant number of outreach activities. During the first two years of the program, nearly 90 activities were completed by participants, reaching over 2,000 individuals across the Region. Table 9.1 provides insight into the reach of the Program over the first two years of the current funding cycle.

Examples of activities completed typical to the program include:

- Teaching public library staff at Hennepin County (MN) Libraries about NLM resources for the public
- Teaching high-school students in the Detroit area how to use freely available NLM resources, such as PubMed and PubMed Central
- Presenting MedlinePlus to seniors at a senior center in North Dakota
- Presenting a session on health information for older adults at a public library in Iowa
- Promoting NLM resources to health professionals at a rural health conference in Indiana

The Program has also been successful in promoting the resources and services of the participating library; the librarian conducting the work becomes a local contact, providing opportunities for activities in the future and elevating the visibility of the participating library. Outreach librarians incorporated within projects funded by the GMR often develop long-term collaborative relationships benefiting both parties. As an example, a librarian from a participating library given the

TABLE 9.1 NNLM portal reporting statistics

Year	Number of Outreach Activities[a]	Number of Participants Reached
2016–2017	24	630
2017–2018	64	1,386
Totals	88	2,016

a Outreach activities are defined as trainings, presentations, or site visit to a current or potential Network member.

opportunity to present at a senior center on behalf of the office was then included in future programming at the center, establishing an ongoing partnership.

POLs provide the GMR with feedback from participants in their programs. Many participants are unaware of the availability of these free, quality resources from NLM. Train-the-trainer programs, such as training public librarians how to access consumer information online, extend the Program's reach further. POLs share resources with teachers who in turn integrate them in lesson plans. Some POLs author articles for state-wide library association newsletters, informing public librarians about easy-to-use resources.

Lessons learned

The biggest roadblock to the revised program was introducing and transitioning to a funding model under which all participating libraries could operate. When stipends to libraries were no longer possible, the office first introduced the option of applying for subawards from the funded GMR grant as a financial model for the program. A subaward is an award with a fixed budget which is tied to a detailed project plan, submitted by the applicant. Subawards are intended for a project to take place over a fixed period of time, or period of performance, and are to meet predetermined objectives. Feedback was that the subaward model did not allow for the flexibility needed for outreach activities throughout the year. Outreach opportunities often arise unplanned, and the subaward model did not allow for making changes to the approved plan frequently or easily. Next, the current pay-for-performance model was introduced, in which participating libraries took part in activities as they came up throughout the year and invoiced the office for each activity. There were challenges in transitioning all of the partners to the new model, and several required additional documentation in the form of a signed agreement from purchasing divisions. Ultimately, all participants were successful in transitioning to the current model at their institution.

Upon the transition to a new funding model, participating libraries required support with the invoicing process, which was not previously an element to the program. Under the new model, those performing outreach were required to track expenses related to a particular outreach activity in order to submit an invoice for reimbursement. Formerly, with the annual stipend, invoices were processed once at the end of the contract year and were not itemized. The Network Librarian supports participating libraries with the process and has developed tools within the guide to make participation as easy as possible. One tool is a set of invoice templates, which had to be reworked for clarity, and the addition of estimated costs on the proposed partner outreach activity form. The transition was successful, but there was a heavier workload for all parties involved during and immediately after the change in funding model.

One key to the success of the program has been communication with the partner library, administrators, finance departments, accountants, GMR staff, and designated outreach librarians doing the work. In several instances, GMR staff were required to meet with participating outreach libraries and their finance staff to resolve issues. The librarian performing outreach was included on all communications, from the identification of the potential activity through reimbursement. The Network Librarian is at the ready to respond to any questions from the POLs and make adjustments throughout the process; For example, the process flowchart was updated as the process evolved and additional resources (links) were added when requested by POLs. The relationships that developed between personnel at the participating library and the Network Librarian proved to be an essential component to the program.

Communication included guidance on whether or not a particular outreach event is appropriate to undertake on behalf of the GMR office. For example, outreach traditionally performed by the library as part of its own mission may not be appropriate if the intent is to serve the library's own faculty and students. However, activities to reach health professionals, educators, or librarians who are not affiliated with their institution is within the scope of the program, particularly if the outreach includes promotion of or training on NLM resources. Outreach to the public is included within the scope of both partner organizations. The Program benefits both partners, linking the partner library with potential future outreach opportunities and supporting the library in the projects that the POL has identified.

The Network Evaluation Office (NEO), an office of NNLM, created evaluation tools for training activities –including those performed by external trainers such as the outreach librarians in the Program. Trainers administer an evaluation at completion of activities and submit the responses to NNLM electronically. Of respondents for the 13 POL activities for which data was collected (N = 118 respondents), 97% responded that they had learned about a new resource; 96% reported learning a new skill; 92% agreed or strongly agreed that their ability to find appropriate information was improved; 93% of participants agreed or strongly agreed that they would start using a new resource as a result of the training; and 89% indicated that they agreed or strongly agreed that they would tell others about a resource they learned as a result of training. One challenge of the Program is illustrating an accurate picture of the impact that the combined outreach activities have on the public. In the future, existing evaluation data for individual activities may be combined with qualitative data from participating outreach librarians to provide a more accurate picture of the overall impact of the Program.

Reproducibility

Implementation of a project similar to the Partner Outreach Library Program might involve a group of academic health sciences libraries within a state combining and coordinating outreach efforts in a similar manner. Such coordination could reduce duplication and leverage limited outreach resources, including personnel time and travel costs. A network like this might undertake similar projects in order to extend the reach of their services to the public through activities at community centers or other community-based organizations. Another possibility could be a program developed as a partnership between a state public health department and an academic library, through which the partners could create and implement health information interventions involving health sciences librarians.

Libraries considering a similar project should look to develop partnerships with institutions that share a common mission. In the context of the Partner Outreach Library Project, this meant locating libraries that share a mission of outreach with NNLM and have designated resources, in the form of personnel time, to conduct outreach within the state. Finally, any partnership of this nature is dependent upon consistent communication between parties. Communication was particularly important during the redesign of this program, but ongoing communication is the most important element to program maintenance. It is necessary to share changes to NLM resources (databases discontinued, combined, or new resources launched), and also to communicate information about ongoing and upcoming initiatives. This information allows participants in the program to select appropriate audiences and venues for outreach work that address the priorities of all partners involved in the collaboration.

The authors would like to thank the National Library of Medicine and the National Network of Libraries of Medicine National Coordinating Office for affording the GMR the opportunity to fund these exciting partnerships and especially the dedicated professional health sciences librarians who are essential to the success of the program (Figures 9.3 and 9.4).

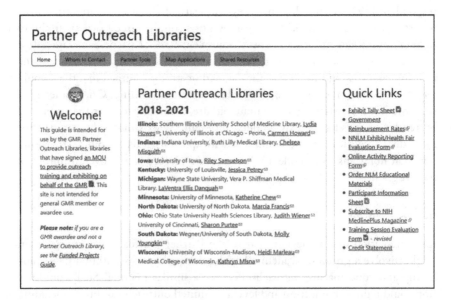

FIGURE 9.3 Partner Outreach Libraries guide landing page.

MEMORANDUM OF UNDERSTANDING

The [Institution] agrees to serve as a Partner Outreach Library for the National Network of Libraries of Medicine (NNLM) Greater Midwest Region (GMR) from May 1, 2018 – April 30, 2021. NNLM GMR is funded through the National Library of Medicine, National Institutes of Health, and Department of Health and Human Services under Grant Number 1UG4LM012346 with The University of Iowa. A successful partner Outreach Library exhibits the following criteria:

- A mission of health information outreach to the community
- Qualified health information professionals with time dedicated to outreach activities
- An NNLM member
- Familiarity with NLM/NIH resources

Under this agreement, the National Network of Libraries of Medicine (NNLM), Greater Midwest Region (GMR) office will:

- Reimburse partner libraries for outreach events, such as providing instruction or exhibiting, on behalf of the GMR*
- Reimburse mileage, lodging, and meals up to the federal government rate (www.gsa.gov) for traveling on behalf of the GMR
- Reimburse partner libraries for incidental expenses, such as printing materials, postage, parking, shipping, or other related costs
- Reimburse partner libraries for the cost of preparing for and hosting up to two National Library of Medicine traveling exhibitions each year
- Provide support for outreach opportunities within their state
- Coordinate quarterly meetings for partner outreach librarians

*Personnel time for activities will be reimbursed at the institution's hourly rate or a flat rate of $300 per event, as negotiated.

Under this agreement, the Partner Outreach Library will:

- Perform outreach in their state to groups unaffiliated with their institution
- Communicate with the GMR office prior to teaching or exhibiting on behalf of the office
- Stay current with NLM/NIH resources
- Follow reporting procedures for events as outlined by NLM
- Submit invoices for reimbursement to the GMR office, minimally quarterly each year

Partner libraries may withdraw at any time during the agreement period (May 1, 2018 – April 30, 2021) by giving written notice to GMR at which time GMR will no longer reimburse that institution for outreach. The Greater Midwest Region will continue to fund activities during the agreement period until funds budgeted for these activities are expended. Indirect costs (F&A) are not eligible for activities under this agreement.

The Partner Outreach Library Program is intended to fund small outreach events within the library's state. Program participants are encouraged to apply for awards (https://nnlm.gov/gmr/funding) for projects that fall beyond the scope of this agreement.

FIGURE 9.4 Memorandum of understanding.

Notes

1 NNLM membership is on an institutional level. Any library, institution, or organization which has health information access as part of its mission is available for membership. Membership in the Network is free.
2 The GMR consists of the ten states of Illinois, Indiana, Iowa, Kentucky, Michigan, Minnesota, North Dakota, Ohio, South Dakota, and Wisconsin.
3 The SCR RML was then located at the Texas Medical Center in Houston, TX. The SCR consists of the states of Arkansas, Louisiana, New Mexico, Oklahoma, and Texas. As of the 2016–2021 grant period, the SCR RML is based in Fort Worth, TX, at the University of North Texas Health Science Center.
4 https://www.nlm.nih.gov/hmd/about/exhibition/

References

Bunting, A. (1987). The nation's health information network: History of the regional medical library program, 1965–1985. *Bulletin of the Medical Library Association, 75*(3 Suppl), 1–62.

National Network of Libraries of Medicine. (2018). About NNLM. Retrieved from https://nnlm.gov

SECTION B
Education

10

INTRODUCTION

Libraries addressing the educational needs of the community

Henry R. Cunningham

Education is of upmost importance to everyone, whether a child in school or an adult. We are constantly learning new things and have an urge to learn and build on previous knowledge as we broaden our horizons. New knowledge may be gained from multiple sources, including books, the media, social media, and churches, among others. While schools may be the primary source of education for children, this is not the case for adults who are no longer in school, who may need to explore alternative avenues for information and knowledge. While accessibility to new knowledge may be quite easy for those with financial resources, it may be a challenge for those from low-income households. Where then can these individuals go to access new information? One answer may be the community library.

Libraries have played a major role in communities, both urban and rural, serving as a place to borrow books and movies, read, study, or even make copies of documents, among others. For decades libraries have been serving in these roles, sometimes even as a place for friends to socialize. However, with increasing demands in communities, particularly in low-income communities, public libraries are seeing their traditional role change. Libraries are increasingly called upon to provide critical educational services to their communities (American Library Association, 2018) as they attempt to address the needs in their communities. To a large extent, much learning is taking place outside of the formal setting and occurring instead in libraries. As a result, public libraries are transforming their traditional role and increasing their services to include education and necessary life skills (Erich, 2018). These are skills necessary in everyday life activities. Some of these services are conducted alone, while in some cases libraries are required to collaborate with other entities such as colleges and universities to provide the needed services to their communities.

This section of the book will explore several ways in which libraries collaborated with other entities to address critical community needs. These collaborations were done in an effort to better educate and inform individuals on certain issues of importance. These chapters share models of how public libraries collaborated with other stakeholders to provide certain community services that are outside of the traditional role of public libraries.

Harhai discussed "Engaged, Educated and Entertained: Employing a Facilitated Discussion Model" where a model called facilitated discussion, utilized by the public library to teach literacy skills to community members, is presented. The model used books, videos, and facilitators who are knowledgeable about selected topics to enhance literacy. These literacy projects were undertaken to increase and enhance literacy development in the community. The use of books, videos and expert speakers were used to explore various topics such as the World War 1. Another project explored science, technology, engineering, and math (STEM) topics in an effort to interest and educate adults on science topics. The objectives of these projects were to inform adults in the community about various topics while enhancing literacy.

A summer book club is the focus of Barrera, Skinner, and Reilly's work in "The Carver Cubs Summer Book Club: A Reciprocal Collaboration Between a Neighborhood Library and a Graduate Elementary Teacher Preparation Program". The program discusses a partnership between a public library and the graduate teacher preparation program at Louisiana State University in the United States. The program is about a service-learning or community-based learning course, whereby education students from the university participated in the summer program as part of the course requirement. Students assisted with a reading-intensive program, which greatly increased exposure to literature and reading and comprehension for the children participating in the summer camp. This program is a true partnership that is mutually beneficial. It provided an opportunity for pre-service teachers to gain hands-on experience in teaching and working with a diverse learning group, while for the children in the summer camp, they were provided with free instruction in reading through group and individual instruction.

Russo in "Information Literacy Through Service-Learning" provided a similar program on how libraries are engaged in service-learning or community-based learning courses to enhance literacy. Students from Louisiana State University in the United States were assigned to a local public library as part of their course. Their role was to provide assistance to the library staff in various capacity, thus familiarizing them with services the library has to offer and how these services were carried out. Library staff received much needed assistance in getting the work of the library done, while students were exposed to a wealth of electronic and print material within the library that is at their disposal.

Another project presented to educate the community is that of a monthly health talk. Kang, Mancini, Raivich and Wong in "The Monthly Health Talk: How a

Consumer Health Library Became a Hub for a Successful health Education Event Through Partnerships and Community Engagement", present a project that is a collaboration among several entities to provide monthly health presentations to members of the community to educate participants on health-related topics. Knowledgeable individuals present the topics covered in an attempt to address prevention, safety, wellness, and self-management. What is unique about this particular project is that participants come from different linguistic background, many of whom do not speak or understand English. To address this issue, interpreters are provided at the sessions, enabling non-English speakers to benefit from these monthly talks.

The authors spent quite a bit of time discussing how the collaboration was developed and what drove them to seek out partners to address the identified need. For those interested in similar collaborations, this section provides strategies on how to develop partnerships and with whom to develop these partnerships. They explored the mutual interest that existed between and among the various stakeholders that drove them to collaborate. The systematic approach taken to develop the project should also prove helpful for others as the authors went into detail to outline the steps taken as these projects were developed. The level of detail provided ensures that anyone who wants to replicate a program of this nature has somewhat of a template onto which one can build in creating their own initiative.

This section also covers the challenges in developing these models to educate the community, as they were all new programs that originated through joint interest from the various stakeholders. The authors however, did a great job discussing how they were able to address the challenges faced and the lessons learned from the process. This section should be particularly helpful for individuals or entities interested in developing similar programs in their community so as to avoid the pitfalls encountered in these projects.

These models presented provide varied opportunities in which libraries may collaborate with other stakeholders to address critical educational needs in the community. It speaks to the changing roles of libraries that demonstrate the need for libraries to be more proactive in serving their communities in ways that go beyond merely a place to borrow and read a book. This is a new role for many libraries and librarians but one for which they seem poised to embrace in their community.

References

American Library Association. (2018). Let's talk about it. Retrieved from http://www.ala.org/tools/programming/ltai

Erich, A. (2018). The role of public libraries in non-formal learning. *Romanian Journal for Multidimensional Education, 10*(3), 17–24. doi:10.18662/rrem/59

11

INFORMATION LITERACY THROUGH SERVICE-LEARNING

Michael F. Russo

LSU and LSU libraries

Louisiana State University (LSU) is among 1% of universities in the United States designated a land-, sea-, and space-grant institution. LSU educates roughly 30,000 young men and women of all ethnic, religious, and cultural backgrounds each academic year (LSU Office of Finance & Administration, 2019, University Fall Facts 2018). As stated in LSU's Strategic Plan 2025, the University exists to address "the broader needs of society" (LSU Office of Academic Affairs, 2017, p. 1).

LSU's footprint in Baton Rouge is enormous. The campus is situated on 2,130 acres south of downtown Baton Rouge (Ruffin et al., 2006, p. 49). As a corporate citizen of the greater metropolitan area, the University recognizes the reciprocal relationship between University and community and its obligation to the community and is therefore committed to public service in many areas affecting the progress and wellbeing of the larger local community.

The LSU Libraries exists to "advance research, teaching, and learning across every discipline" (LSU Libraries, 2018, para. About Us). In addition to supporting the work of students and faculty in addressing the broader needs of society, as a publicly funded entity the Libraries also serves the general public, providing research and reference services and allowing check-out of certain library materials with the presentation of official state identification. In addition to providing millions of books, hundreds of databases, and individual and collaborative study spaces, the Libraries provides its core constituencies with expertise in subject-specific research and with education to help them take advantage of the Libraries' many resources.

Information literacy (IL)

Library and Information Science is a discipline, which exists in the service of information and the information user. For decades, LSU Libraries has engaged in bibliographic instruction of one kind or another. Library instruction has occurred and still occurs on many levels:

- Individual, point-of-service instruction takes place daily at the Reference Desk. Librarians explain the following to student-scholars; the mechanics of research, how to use specific databases, and how to employ strings of keywords to get focused results, thus equipping them to move forward on their own.
- Librarians also provide extended one-on-one research assistance to students and faculty. By appointment, librarians will interview patrons to determine exactly what they need to know, and then guide them in the use of appropriate research tools. These consultations last as long as necessary and occur as often as necessary to achieve results for the patron.
- Librarians also meet with classes during the semester, generally on a one-time basis but more often if needed. These one-time instruction sessions are requested by faculty to prepare their classes for up-coming research papers.

The Libraries, until recently, offered a one-credit course called Research Methods and Materials, more commonly referred to as LIS 1001. LIS 1001 was designed to educate undergraduates in the use of specific library resources to enable them to complete their research assignments. The LIS 1001 course was about the nature of Information – the different kinds, levels, and depths of information; how it is created, organized, and stored; how to search for and find it; and how to use it. The challenge of teaching LIS 1001 online and in the classroom has been getting the students to see that the skills they learned were not just for this course, but were transferrable to their other courses and to their lives outside academia. Librarian-instructors want students to understand that the need and search for information were things that would be in their lives always and that if they understood something of information they would be the better for it.

The Center for Community Engagement, Learning, and Leadership (CCELL)

One important element of LSU's community relations effort is the Center for Community Engagement, Learning, and Leadership (CCELL). CCELL was established specifically to promote "the integration of teaching, research, and service to encourage civic responsibility and to enhance learning and social accountability" (LSU CCELL, para. About Us). CCELL does this by actively cultivating campus and community partnerships. The point of CCELL is not to supply volunteers to community programs – that is done by another program.

The CCELL program's focus is to combine instruction with service to enhance the student instruction and connect the students directly and intimately to their community partners. Even as the community partner benefits through the free services the students provide, the students also benefit by applying what they are taught in the classroom to real-world situations. The knowledge they acquire in the classroom becomes something real and connected to their environment. Depending on how the classroom teacher and the community partner structure the experience, this approach can be an all-around win.

The origin of the idea

The resources available through the CCELL were integral in transforming the LIS 1001 course and in reaching out to the community. Since the instruction in the original course was focused specifically on LSU Libraries' resources, services, organization, and how to use them, it was identified that lessons would be more beneficial if students experienced working in a library themselves, interacting with people who needed help finding information. Students potentially would benefit even more from service in a public library than in an academic library. The rationale for using a public library setting was once students graduated from the University, they would more likely go to a local public library for information; and there would be public libraries pretty much wherever they might relocate. If they were familiar with one, they would likely be familiar with all. Thus, this service-learning course would include partnership with the Carver Branch of the East Baton Rouge Parish Public Library (Carver), chosen because of its proximity to the University.

The course would have to be radically re-designed, agreement would have to be formalized with Carver, and all this would have to be accomplished before getting approval for the service-learning designation for the course so the students could earn service-learning credit from the University. Once this process was in motion, it took nearly a year to get to the point of actually putting the revised course on the schedule.

Training

Faculty new to the service-learning program took a semester-long course of instruction from the CCELL staff. Teachers learned the basic philosophy of service-learning and heard from faculty and community partners who have participated in the program. Faculty learned about several projects in which other faculty members partnered with community stakeholders for service-learning courses. These include how a Biological Engineering class partnered with an elementary school to build a new playground, a bike shop owner who taught low-income children how to build and maintain bicycles through his partnership with a Mechanical Engineering class. The coordinator of the Volunteers in Public Schools program also spoke of his partnership with an Education class, which furnished reading tutors for children with learning difficulties. The presenters emphasized two things: (1) the activities in which the students engaged should be mutually beneficial to the community partner and the student and not simply busy work; and (2) the work the students did should be an integral part of their instruction, meaning it should relate directly to what they were being taught in the classroom.

Faculty preparing to teach service-learning courses got a lot of practice creating goals, assignments, and rubrics so they could accurately measure their students' performance. The final project was a course syllabus, which others in the class critiqued.

The community partner: consultations and needs

CCELL staff made initial contact with Carver. Several discussions with the manager and supporting personnel of the Carver Branch were held. The Branch Head was immediately agreeable to the project and was ready to collaborate. He had had considerable experience working with students from other LSU service-learning classes, but never with students from a Library Science class. This would be the first time Carver had received the benefit of students who were actually studying the organization and function of information and libraries. The public librarians were quite enthusiastic.

Each neighborhood library is a reflection of the unique neighborhood it serves. The Carver Branch serves a lower income, urban neighborhood. The needs of Carver's patrons, the students would discover, were characteristic of the neighborhood's socio-economic status. Unlike the usual inquiries for information on humanities or scientific topics that occur in the LSU library, inquiries in Carver were for practical information. Many patrons needed help accessing the Internet in order to complete requirements for government assistance or to submit job applications. Some needed to download and print forms and other documents. Occasionally, neighborhood students needed guidance to information for school projects.

Through direct observation and hours spent at the Information Desk with Carver staff, the patrons' needs became apparent. Additionally, through email exchanges with the Adult Services Librarian and the Branch Head, the service aspect of the course slowly evolved.

Design of the course: objectives

The overall goals of LIS 1001 have always been for students to be able to recognize when they need information, know where to find it, how to evaluate it, and how to use it effectively. These are the main ideas behind the concept of Information Literacy. In order to achieve these goals, students must have a basic understanding of the research process as well as the organization and retrieval of library materials. The intent of the course has always been to expose students to a variety of print and electronic material and to ingrain in them the knowledge that the library is a repository of useful information to which they have access. Through this new iteration of the course, students would recognize the fact that, though University and Public Libraries serve their particular communities in different ways and with different resources, both do this with information.

The result of discussions with the Carver librarians was a short list of specific things the library needed which they felt the students could do:

- Students would "shadow" at the Information Desk. Staff did not feel the students should interact with patrons on their own, feeling that librarian supervision was necessary. For the most part, students would see what the patrons needed and how the Carver staff was addressing those needs. Just seeing the range of queries and their nature would be revelatory in terms of how dependent the community is on the library.
- Students would be allowed to assist patrons with computer problems, with supervision by the library staff. The students had enough general computer skills to allow them to address many of the problems less computer literate patrons would encounter.
- They could also shelf-read. The purpose of shelf reading is to make sure books are in proper call number order on the shelves, making them findable by the patrons. Having students perform this essential task would give them a solid understanding of the subject categorization that is the basis for the Dewey Decimal Classification scheme and, hopefully, have the side effect of revealing the value of shelf browsing.
- Students would be allowed to process discarded material, which would require them to become familiar with the library catalog, a fundamental tool when doing library research.
- Finally, the students would also evaluate the appropriateness of donations to the library of used books and other materials. Students would get further experience using the catalog as well as evaluating material (an essential element in Information Literacy) and they would necessarily become familiar with the Collection Development Policy, giving them some grounding in the decision-making process of the library.

To help students become familiar with the library they would be serving, Carver's Branch Head agreed to issue library cards to all students in the course.

The course

The course began with an orientation session at the Carver library. Before students began their service, they were introduced to the people they would be working with and to the place where they would be working. At this stage, the importance of showing up was emphasized. The students were to understand that the hours they signed up to work in the library represented a commitment equal to being present for any job for which they were paid. Absences would be reported by the Carver staff and would result in a lower grade.

By way of a sign-up sheet, students chose the hours they would work; since the course lasted only seven weeks, they worked only five hours spread over the seven weeks. After each service hour, students were required to submit a narrative reflection, which was to be more than a mere description of what happened while they were at the library. The reflection was to be a thoughtful rumination on the meaning and impact of their overall experience performing service. This reflection is an essential element of the service-learning experience. As such, the reflections represented the majority of the course grade. A list of prompts in the form of questions was provided to give students ideas about what they should address in their reflections. Some examples of those prompts:

- What issue was addressed?
- What job or service was performed?
- What was your overall impression of the patron being served?
- Can you relate your experience to anything you have learned so far in class?
- What did you learn from the service experience? What would you have liked to learn?
- Has your view of the community or the community partner changed? If so, how has it changed and what changed it? If not, what is your view?

A rubric explaining how the reflections would be scored was also provided (see Table 11.1). According to the rubric, to rate the highest level (Distinguished), a reflection had to demonstrate awareness of the purpose of service, apply course concepts to the service provided, acknowledge responsibility to the community, show the experience had some impact on the student's personal life, and display evidence of clear critical thinking overall.

The course was structured to include all the concepts and skills normally taught in LIS 1001, but structured in a way that the teaching of particular ideas coincided with what the students would be doing at the Carver library. For example, library organizational schemes are taught in every section of LIS 1001. It is important for every library user to understand a library's organizational scheme in order for the library experience to be successful. Thus, we teach our students about the Library of Congress and Dewey Decimal Classification systems as well as others. This instruction took place at the time the students were to begin shelf reading. When the time came for the students to evaluate discards and gifts, evaluation as a key information literacy concept was taught.

Inasmuch as the overall goals of the course were to get students to understand the nature of information and that seeking it would be a lifelong activity, applying their classroom instruction by using it to serve others in pursuit of information would, reinforce those lessons to become a permanent home in their skill sets.

TABLE 11.1 Student evaluation

	Distinguished (4)	Proficient (3)	Apprentice (2)	Novice (1)	Comments (0)
Awareness of purpose of service [civic engagement] – 18%	Student understands complexity of both issues and solutions as well as his/her personal role in solutions.	Student demonstrates understanding of the complexity of the community's issues and possible solutions.	Student expresses some awareness of community's issues	Student demonstrates limited awareness of community's issues. Does not go beyond description of activities.	
Application of course concepts to service-learning [academics] – 18%	Student uses service experience to evaluate course concepts and effectiveness of service.	Student demonstrates a clear understanding of the relationship between course concepts and service experience.	Student expresses some connection between course concepts and service experience	Student does not apply course concepts or the connection to service experience is limited/unclear.	
Responsibility to community [civic engagement] – 18%	Student embodies personal sense of responsibility to community regarding issues pertinent to service experience and actively participates in the collective effort to solve these issues.	Student integrates personal sense of responsibility to community regarding issues pertinent to service experience and expresses a commitment to working towards specific solutions.	Student expresses insight into community issues pertinent to the service experience and demonstrates some awareness of personal sense of responsibility.	Student demonstrates limited awareness of personal responsibility to community	

(Continued)

	Distinguished (4)	Proficient (3)	Apprentice (2)	Novice (1)	Comments (0)
Impact on student's personal life [personal growth] – 18%	Student uses changes in perspective to guide choices and behaviors in areas related to service experience as well as in areas related to other social issues.	Student uses changes in perspective to guide choices and behaviors, but only in areas related to service experience	Student expresses connection between service and self; demonstrates empathy and change in attitudes, perspectives, beliefs, or understanding of his/her own skill.	Student expresses a limited connection between service and self. Demonstrates limited empathy and little or no change in attitudes, perspective, beliefs, or behavior.	
Critical thinking [academics] (overall essay) – 18%	Student assesses and evaluates perspectives, knowledge and opinions gained from course concepts and service experience, and links these assessments to own perspectives and opinions on social issues.	Student assesses and evaluates perspectives, knowledge, and opinions gained from course concepts and service experience.	Student asks questions and shows awareness of multiple perspectives. Opinions are stated with some analysis and support	Student accepts things at face value, as if all opinions were created equal. Opinions are stated without analysis or support.	
Mechanics [spelling and grammar; citation] – 10%	Writer makes few errors in grammar or spelling. All sources are accurately documented and correctly formatted.	Writer makes some errors in grammar or spelling. Sources are documented but not correctly formatted.	Writer makes numerous errors in grammar or spelling. Some sources are not accurately documented nor correctly formatted.	Writer demonstrates indifference or incompetence regarding spelling, grammar, and citation of sources.	
Total					

Evaluation of the course

This was the first time LIS 1001 was taught as a service-learning course. It will likely be the only time, despite being successful, because LSU Libraries no longer teaches LIS 1001. LSU librarians agreed with the assessment of authorities – like Steven Bell (2008), Trudi Jacobson and Beth Mark (2000), Owusu-Ansah (2004), and others – that students should see a tangible use for skills being taught. As Jacobson and Mark wrote, "…if students do not immediately apply their information literacy skills to a content-based course assignment, they tend not to recognize the relevance of such skills to other courses" (Jacobson & Mark, 2000, p. 261).

Normally, the course was taught devoid of context, to be taken for one credit or to fill a hole in a student's schedule, but with no obvious use or concrete purpose to give the effort consequence. The question for instructors of LIS 1001 has always been how to make the course relevant, how to give students a full understanding of what they were being taught and why.

It is felt that embedding IL instruction in a discipline course that requires research gives immediate relevance to the instruction, whereby students understand why they need to be able to use the library effectively. All that being said, while there are improvements that could be made should the service-learning version of the course be taught again, it was, overall, successful in that the eyes of the participating students were opened somewhat wider to the challenges of the community they served and the role the public library plays in meeting those challenges.

The nine students in the class each provided a total of five hours of service. Because of the brief time, the students served in the Carver library, and because the level of activity in the library at any given time was unpredictable – sometimes heavy, sometimes light – the direct service opportunities the students encountered were not as plentiful as one would have hoped. Further limiting direct patron encounters was the fact that two days of service were spent on projects that did not require patron contact: shelf reading and gift evaluation. According to the reports the students submitted of their experience, there were 26 specified encounters with individual patrons and an indeterminate number of other encounters as indicated by expressions such as "a lot of people", "teenagers", and "school-aged children". Specifically identified patron encounters included 11 related to finding materials or information and 15 related to help with technology. There was no way to evaluate the effectiveness of the course other than anecdotally from the students. The staff of the library did not respond to a request for feedback post-course, but the clear sense from the students was that they had done something positive for their service partner.

In their final reflections, several students testified that their experience had had a significant impact on them. Here are a few of their statements:

- I really enjoyed helping out and got a sense of worth by being of service to our community.
- [The work] gave me a new and deeper appreciation for the public library, and what their workers do in order to keep their resources available to the community.
- It felt good to know that I am giving back to my community.
- I value this opportunity, because it made me feel more involved in the Baton Rouge community.

The message of **community service** was received clearly, without ambiguity.

The final project for this course was a pathfinder, a brief listing of sources of information on a specific topic. There were two points to this project. One was to get the students to pull together the various skills and concepts they had learned in the course. This meant they had to be able to find information by using the catalog, databases, and Internet; they had to evaluate the information for its relevance and quality; and they had to present the information in a form that was easy to use and made sense. Pathfinders were formatted as tri-fold brochures and, since these brochures were being offered to the Carver library for use by its patrons, they had to include only material available through the public library.

Topics for these pathfinder brochures were suggested by the Carver library staff, based on the most frequently requested information and the diversity of the Carver community's interests. Students were able to provide lists of publicly available sources for such diverse topics as Louisiana travel, Mardi Gras, scholarships, argumentative essay writing, human trafficking, 3-D printing, and others.

The students came away from this experiment not just with research skills, but with an appreciation of what it means to be an active member of a community. They know now – if they did not already know – that communities are groups of different people, diverse in their beliefs, language, dress, and status, but common in their need to thrive. They came away understanding that the need to thrive is satisfied when there are aid and cooperation and the willingness to reach beyond oneself.

One student wrote of her experience culling gift books this way:

> One [book] that I reviewed is the *Pokémon Deluxe Essential Handbook*. I recommended that this book…be added to Carver's collection because of the increasing interest in Pokémon…as a result of the new app, Pokémon Go. Another book I reviewed was a copy of the King James Version of the *Holy Bible*. The bible was completely worn. The binding was almost completely destroyed. There was evidence of food stains and evidence that something was spilled on the pages. I put this book in the discard section because it was not in good enough condition to be added to Carver's collection.

And another student described the end of her service as "bittersweet".

As reported by students, the Carver staff appreciated the work the students, such as the one quoted above, did. To cite just one other instance, a student assigned to organize and re-shelve music CDs discovered an error in the labeling of some of them and pointed this out to the supervising librarian. The student reported, "The librarian really appreciated it because it was not correct and needed to be changed".

Challenges and going forward

The service-learning program at LSU continues. Despite the discontinuation of LIS 1001 as a stand-alone course, information literacy instruction continues as well. Today, subject librarians collaborate with professors in those disciplines for which the librarians have collection development responsibility to provide the research instruction students need to complete class assignments. This is an IL instruction model that can be applied to any course, even one with a service-learning component.

By collaborating with a service-learning course, librarians can make themselves part of the service process while simultaneously imparting the essential information literacy skills necessary to do college-level research. Thus, it will be as necessary for the librarian to become familiar with the community partner's needs as it will be for the students. In this way, the academic library will become an important resource to the community partner and the community at large, as well as to the students.

As well organized as the course was, there absolutely are changes and improvements that could make the course even more effective. For example, Carver staff discouraged the students who took the course from directly assisting patrons seeking information, though, as mentioned above, some direct interactions did occur. Students were limited to simply observing the transaction with the librarian on duty. To provide the students with a more meaningful and hands-on experience, a script to use during such a transaction and classroom practice with the script could be added to their preparation for service.

Though the students' reflection papers fulfilled basic requirements, the papers could have been deeper in terms of how the students' service was perceived and how they themselves had changed (or not) because of their service. More specific guidelines and possibly examples of excellent and poor reflection papers would lead the students to produce reflections that are more ruminative.

Class discussions of students' service experiences should be included to explore their perceptions and misgivings. Discussions during and after the course with the community partner's staff should be added for the same reasons.

The library is already integral to the campus community. Stepping even a short distance off campus can link a University Library to the community it and the University's graduates will ultimately serve.

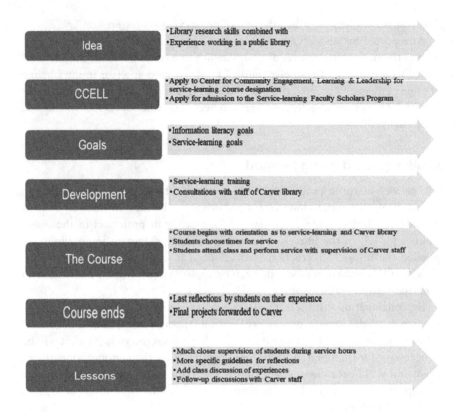

FIGURE 11.1 Flow chart of development and activities for LIS 1001 service-learning.

References

Bell, S. (2008, November 25). IL course credit does not equal credibility. Retrieved from ACRLog: https://acrlog.org/2008/11/25/il-course-credit-does-not-equal-credibility/

Jacobson, T., & Mark, B. T. (2000). Separating wheat from chaff: Helping first-year students become information savvy. *The Journal of General Education, 4*, 256. doi:10.1353/jge.2000.0029

LSU Center for Community Engagement, Learning & Leadership (CCELL) web site (n.d.). Retrieved from http://www.lsu.edu/academicaffairs/ccell/about_ccell/who_we_are.php

LSU Libraries. (2018). About the libraries. Retrieved from https://www.lib.lsu.edu/about

LSU Office of Academic Affairs. (2017). LSU strategic plan 2025. Retrieved from http://strategicplan.lsu.edu/

LSU Office of Finance & Administration—Budget & Planning. (2019). University fall facts 2018. Retrieved from https://www.lsu.edu/bgtplan/facts/pdfs/2018fallfacts_final.pdf

Owusu-Ansah, E. (2004). Information literacy and higher education: Placing the academic library in the center of a comprehensive solution. *Journal of Academic Librarianship, 30*(1), 3–16. Retrieved from http://libezp.lib.lsu.edu/login?url=https://search.ebscohost.com/login.aspx?direct=true&db=edswss&AN=000220076300002&site=eds-live&scope=site&profile=eds-main

Ruffin, T. F., Jackson, J., & Hebert, M. J. (2006). *Under stately oaks: A pictorial history of LSU.* Baton Rouge: Louisiana State University Press.

12

ENGAGED, EDUCATED, AND ENTERTAINED

Employing a facilitated discussion model

Marilyn Harhai

A facilitated discussion can serve as a framework for libraries looking to involve professional, community, and service organizations in literacy projects. Book discussions are a tried and true programming staple in libraries (Hooper, 2016). While at first blush, the possibilities of expanding the book discussion model to foster health, wellbeing, and quality of life outcomes of diverse populations in a variety of settings may not be obvious; however, growing the model to foster literacy development and to incorporate community engagement is an organic process. The facilitated discussion model consists of books, videos, and expert facilitators on selected topics. With its foundation of libraries, books, and community experts, the model is ideal to foster literacy. The facilitated discussion model is scalable making it a great starter project with room for growth. The model is described along with several literacy-based projects that were undertaken using this approach and further ideas for expanding the model for literacy development involving the community. Topics can vary based on need and available partners. Participants of any age can use the method for any outcome by using different books, videos, facilitators, and varied community partners.

The library or the community partners can be the source for literacy topics. The reasons libraries provide programming, as explained by the Public Programs Office of the American Library Association, include:

> Libraries are many things to their communities. They offer the practical information people need to improve their quality of life and to increase individual options in a complex society—information about health, education, business, childcare, computers, the environment, looking for a job... and much more.
>
> Libraries also give their communities something less tangible, yet just as essential to a satisfying and productive life—nourishment for the spirit.

Programs in the humanities and the arts that encourage people to think and talk about ethics and values, history, art, poetry, and other cultures are integral to the library's mission.

Such programs help to illuminate the experiences, beliefs and values that unite us as human beings. They stimulate us to make connections where we noticed none before—between our ancestors and ourselves, between one culture and another, between the community and the individual.

(Office of Public Programming, American Library Association,
2018, "Why Should," para. 1–3)

From that list of roles, which libraries can fulfill with programming, it is easy to see that collaborations with numerous community partners addressing a myriad of literacy topics and outcomes are possible. A Pew Research Study found that six in ten Americans say it is "very important" for public libraries to provide free events and activities (Zickuhr et al., 2013, "Free events and activities," para. 1). In the same study, librarians noted that they enjoyed partnering with other local institutions and organizations to expand the types of activities they could offer (para. 4). The facilitated discussion model is adaptable to different partners and literacy topics.

The facilitated discussion model

The facilitated discussion model has early roots in the Let's Talk about It book club discussion series:

A well-established program model for book discussion series is Let's Talk about It, based on a model developed by the Vermont Humanities Council in the 1970s and launched nationally by the American Library Association in the early 1980s, with the support of the National Endowment for the Humanities. This model focuses on reading a common series of texts, chosen by a nationally known scholar, and discussing them in the context of a larger theme. Over the past twenty years, the model has been adopted— and adapted— by hundreds of libraries throughout the country.

(Robinson, 2005, p. 43)

Let's Talk about It includes book selections and expert facilitators (American Library Association, 2018). Library programming using videos and other media also has a long tradition including such events as the Public Broadcasting Service (PBS) series screenings and discussions (Robinson, 2005). Combining books, media, and facilitated discussion integrates these approaches.

The facilitated discussion model evolved using the basic format from a proscribed series into a fluid template. The initial project undertaken with one local library began with a National Science Foundation (NSF) grant called Pushing the Limits (Schwartz, 2012). Pushing the Limits involves fiction books, videos, and facilitated discussion programs to support community consideration of science topics to develop literacy skills (Pushing the Limits, 2017). The concept of using books, experts, and videos to explore community topics was expanded to a number of literacy projects with the library. One discussion series explored the Pennsylvania Library Association's literacy initiative PA Forward, which targets basic, information, civic, financial, and health literacies (Pennsylvania Library Association, 2018). Another group of events, Remembering the Great War: A Film/Book Discussion Series, used the model to commemorate the World War I centenary targeting civic literacy (Maccaferri, 2017). Additionally, topics on diversity, self-improvement, cultural awareness, and others were explored incorporating this model to good effect. Each project was based on a format derived from the Pushing the Limits project.

The seed project, Pushing the Limits, is a packaged science, technology, engineering, and math (STEM) series designed to interest adults in science topics and to expand literacy skills in exploring science. This series has four sessions: Pushing the Limits – Knowledge; Pushing the Limits – Connection; Pushing the Limits – Survival; and Pushing the Limits – Nature (Pushing the Limits, n.d.). The programs are designed around a fiction book and include videos both on the topic and of interviews with the authors of the books. Each session involves viewing the videos and a discussion of the book moderated by a science partner. The science partner is an important component allowing for in-depth discussion of the topics. The science partner also leads the participants to develop their ability to efficiently locate, accurately evaluate, and effectively use information in learning about science. As examples, the book for the connection topic was *Thunderstruck* by Erik Larson (2006) which involved development of the wireless telegraph using a physics professor as the science partner. The book for another topic was *The Land of Painted Caves* by Jean Auel (2011) for which an anthropology professor was tapped. The structure incorporating a book discussion, the use of videos, and experts was used and expanded upon for new projects.

The next events at the local public library, based on the Pennsylvania Library Association initiative PA Forward, used the same basic structure to explore literacy topics, which lent themselves to greatly expanding the use of community partners beyond the science partners. The PA Forward program's foundation is information literacy to help people live healthy, productive lives (Pennsylvania Library Association, 2018). PA Forward defined five essential literacies:

1. Basic Literacy – Libraries can push Pennsylvania to achieve one of the highest literacy rates in the country, a trained and skilled workforce, and a growing economy, tax base, and population.
2. Information Literacy– Libraries can help all Pennsylvanians learn how to use online resources and current technology to improve their education, to enhance their job skills, to develop their personal lives, and to participate fully in a digital society.
3. Civic and Social Literacy – Libraries can play an important role in helping citizens have the knowledge and skills they need to improve their lives, to

participate and contribute effectively to their community, government, and society, and to connect with one another through discourse.

4. Health Literacy – Libraries can play an important role in helping citizens manage their own and their family's wellbeing, and empower them to be effective partners with their healthcare providers so they can live longer, lives that are more productive.

5. Financial Literacy – Libraries can help citizens become informed consumers and guide individuals, small businesses, and other organizations to contribute to the economic vitality of their community through innovation, entrepreneurship, and economic development (Pennsylvania Library Association, n.d.).

Use of the facilitated discussion model to foster health, wellbeing, and quality of life outcomes using the PA Forward information literacies was ideal in generating program ideas and partnerships.

Programming based on the PA Forward topics of financial, health, and civic literacy dovetailed the public library's interests with community organizations that had compatible mandates. Community partners in these areas include banks, financial service providers, insurance agencies, hospitals, healthcare agencies, local government representatives, social service agencies, social clubs, scouting groups, restaurants, other libraries, schools, and colleges. Only the community and topic bound the potential partners.

As the PA Forward topics show, many types of professional organizations, nonprofits, businesses, and educational institutions can participate in the model with the public library toward literacy goals. While the partners and roles vary based on the topics, examples of community involvement demonstrate the range of possibilities.

- College libraries: The university library provided books, staff time, and publicity on the projects. The university library dean supported the projects through the purchase of copies of the books for the university library so that faculty, students, and staff could have easy access. He included the events in the weekly library digital newsletter, and he attended events.

- Community: Community members developed an affinity for some of the programs extending the programs beyond the original projected timeline. They provided food for events and encouraged others to participate.

- High schools: Local schools partnered on topics, provided expert facilitators, and publicized events. Students in relevant programs were encouraged to attend.

- Institutions of higher education: Local colleges provided facilitator expertise on numerous topics. Small amounts of funding were available for projects related to topics of interest to the school. The events were widely publicized in college print and online media. Professors granted students extra credit for attending on-topic programs. Examples of project partners included faculty who were involved in many of the projects. One of the lead project managers was a professor in a library science program. She wrote grants, solicited community partners, handled logistics, selected books and videos, and attended all events. A graduate assistant was able to participate in the project and he gained valuable experience in planning and running events and was able to present a poster session on the Pushing the Limits programs.

- Media: Print and radio media were very generous in covering the events.
- Public library: The local public library provided staff, meeting space, books, publicity, and other support. The public library director wrote and placed media copy, supplied books and videos, allocated space and staff help, collaborated on grants, and attended all events.
- Retail and food establishments in the community: Businesses provided in-kind support (such as donating copies of the books) and publicity. Local restaurants gave discounts on food for events and allowed flyers and posters to be distributed.
- Service organizations in the community: Service agencies in the area were contacted for each topic as it related to their service communities. Agency involvement included financial and in-kind support, experts for the discussions, and publicity. Examples include military veteran service organizations for support of the World War I commemorative project, health agencies on the health literacy topics, and banks and financial institutions on the financial literacy topics. The veteran service organizations were extremely helpful by providing funds, food for events, publicizing events to members, allocating meeting space, and providing facilitators with expertise on discussion topics.

The team structure varied and the cohesive element was the two lead project managers (local public library director and a college professor). Other team members, such as members of the university and public library staff, the graduate assistant and others remained constant serving as the core project team. Other community partners only interacted with one of the lead managers. This allowed for a wide variety of community participation without overburdening individual partners.

Community partners can donate funding or in-kind contributions, collaborate on grants, supply the subject expert facilitators, promote and market events, furnish the venue, provide volunteers, suggest topics, and serve as a source for attendees. Ideas for topics and associated community partnerships include:

- Cooking [health literacy][1]: Local restaurants, grocery stores, agricultural retailers
- Diversity [civic and social literacy]: Places of worship, ethnic social clubs and organizations, university diversity offices
- Eating healthy [health literacy]: Farmers' markets, registered dietitians from the local hospital, culinary arts programs

- Exercise [health literacy]: YMCA/YWCA, local parks and recreation facilities, fitness studios and gyms, rehabilitation facilities
- Financial goals [financial literacy]: Banks, investment firms, college professors
- Health goals [health literacy]: Social service agencies; hospitals, health-related organizations such as the American Cancer Society
- Home repairs [information literacy]: Building supply retailers, vocational schools, trade organizations
- Local interest [civic and social literacy]: Historical societies, social clubs, local authors
- Military [civic and social literacy]: Veteran's social clubs and organizations, ROTC, veterans' affairs office
- Social events [civic and social literacy]: Breweries, tourism bureau, Chamber of Commerce
- Summer activities [information literacy]: The local garden club, Audubon Society, Master Gardeners and the County Extension Office
- Travel [information literacy]: Travel agencies and tour operators, local attractions

Barriers and lessons learned

The structure incorporating a book discussion, videos, and experts with expanded community participation was successful in a number of projects. Some adjustments were made depending on the topic. While the original series used only fiction books, later topics used fiction, nonfiction or both to base the discussions. For example, the World War I commemoration series used both fiction and nonfiction titles paired with popular media depiction of the book or subject:

> Barbara Tuchman's *The Guns of August* (1994), was paired with the feature film *The Day that Shook the World*, starring Christopher Plummer (1994).
> Alan Moorhead's *Gallipoli* (2002), was paired with the feature film *Gallipoli*, starring Mel Gibson (2006).
> Humphrey Cobb's *Paths of Glory* (2010), which was the basis for the feature film of the same name starring Kirk Douglas (2006).
>
> *(Maccaferri, 2017)*

Having paired media allowed for greater participation of those who were not able to read the books. *Guns of August,* for example, is over 600 pages long (Tuchman, 1994). Not everyone could make that commitment though many did. Another modification included showing some shorter videos or clips during the discussions as in the Pushing the Limits series, and for others the videos were to be viewed by the participant prior to the discussion owing to time constraints. Along with these modifications, other ideas to enhance the programs including barriers encountered and lessons learned were identified.

It is important to know your community as you select topics and books. Projects can be developed by reaching out to community partners with which the library wishes to develop a relationship. Solicit ideas from them. A number of the topics undertaken were selected because of grant or funding opportunities from partners associated with the projects.

Do not shy away from potentially controversial subjects. One series involved religious topics and the session on Islam came at a time when anti-Muslim rhetoric was prevalent. The session was one of the best attended and liveliest of the series.

Attention should be given to selecting topics along with books and media. The partner librarian is a crucial element in each series. Selecting books and videos that will spur attendance and discussion will drastically impact success as would be expected. A partner librarian with collection development training and experience can select high-quality thematic materials.

One should not be afraid to use a variety of books and videos in each series. Use fiction, nonfiction, popular movies, documentaries, TV series, whatever works for each topic. Mixing it up can help appeal to a wider audience. An attendee who does not read nonfiction may watch the video or read the fiction selections for a given series. For example, the fiction book *The Land of Painted Caves* by Jean Auel (2011) could be paired with the documentary, *Cave of Forgotten Dreams* (Hertzog, 2011).

Having a theme or topic helps to sell the program to community partners, particularly at the time when marketing the events. One series based on this model was held at the beginning of the year and included events tied to common New Year's resolutions (getting finances in order [financial literacy], eating healthy [health literacy], kicking a bad habit/starting a good habit [multiple literacy topics]).

Make it clear that it is a book *and* media *and* expert facilitator series. Some participants are not excited by preconceived ideas of book clubs or lectures. Make the topic paramount in advertising stressing multiple routes to participation.

The greater the community partners involvement, the greater the investment they have in the success of the program. Simply asking for a donation does not generate sufficient buy-in. Some community partners have a large following who will attend the events. Groups such as the local Audubon Society have large memberships who support their events. Using one of their members as a subject expert facilitator can boost attendance.

Another action one may take is to look for partners who benefit from being involved. Often service organizations and community agencies need a venue for outreach. Then it is not just a donation but an active partnership. Look for partners who have similar goals for literacy development.

The more connections to the other areas that a project can generate, the more likely the program will be a success. Health literacy can be tied into college and high-school classes, nursing programs, the local farmers market, restaurants, service clubs, hospitals, and more.

Attention must be given to choosing each discussion leader/expert so it is done carefully. Subject knowledge is important but not as important as being able to stimulate discussion. Be clear that the facilitator is a resource for the discussion not presenting or lecturing. Attendees should direct the course of the conversation.

In an attempt to reach everyone, include videos so those who do not want to or have time to read a book can participate. Taking such actions will help to provide opportunities for everyone to be involved. The model for the project is adaptable. It can support a one-time program on a topic or a series of related sessions. Consider the idea of a year's worth of events held on the same day of the month each in partnership with different community collaborators on different literacy topics.

Consider using various locations beside the public library, depending on the topic. Consider locations relevant to the topic such as service organization facilities, garden centers, social clubs, restaurants, partner facilities, whatever fits the topic. This can draw attention to local partners and can potentially enhance the presentation depending on the topic. Examples would be viewing plants at a garden center, watching a cooking demonstration at a local restaurant, or practicing activities at a recreation center.

It is to be expected that one series or event may not resonate with the target audience despite much thought put into planning. One grant-based project on current military topics was undertaken. The series were planned carefully and marketed widely; however, attendance was spare. The second military-related theme or the WWI centenary programs were so successful that after the original four events described above, an additional four events were scheduled. Keep trying and learn from each experience.

Finally, be creative in looking for community partners and expert facilitators. Not everyone will say yes. Simply talking with members of the community raises the visibility of the library and they may think of the library the next time that they do have a need for literacy programming or an education venue.

In addition to these ideas, there are excellent resources to get started. Irons, *Film Programming for Public Libraries,* gives practical advice for selecting media, equipment and technology needs, and legal issues in using film in the library (2014). As the model makes use of media, this book can provide solid advice on this aspect of the program.

Robertson, *Cultural Programming for Libraries,* includes chapters on collaboration and series, formats, themes, and tie-ins and is a step-by-step guide to planning cultural programming (2005). This book discusses many aspects of putting on a facilitated discussion program.

Use some of the ideas from Table 12.1 for inspiration.

The basic facilitated discussion model combining books, videos, and discussion with a subject expert facilitator can be applied to many settings, partnerships, and literacy topics. Topics geared toward enhancing health and the quality of life can be adapted with excellent results. The model lends itself to incorporating community partners in a variety of roles, which is the basis for numerous

TABLE 12.1 Ideas to get started

How to select...	
Topics	Analyze circulation statistics for popular subjects.
	Ask community partners.
	Generate ideas from grants or funding opportunities.
	Match the topic to the time of the year or holidays.
	Pick a topic that matches available books or subject experts.
	Read the local newspaper for current issues of interest.
	Review national, state, and local library initiatives.
	Start with a packaged event such as Let's Talk about It or Pushing the Limits.
Partners	Brainstorm community groups with mandates in the topic area.
	Consider new initiatives with current partners.
	Consult the library's employees, board of directors, or Friends group for suggestions.
	Look for partners through civic groups such as the Rotary Club or Chamber of Commerce.
Books/videos	Consult with a collection development or readers' advisory librarian.
	Look on the Web for ideas such as *Cooking the Books: Food Programs in Libraries* (NoveList, 2016).
	Refer to finding aids including the ALA Readers' Advisory Series (ALAStore, n.d.).
	Start with what the library already owns.
	Use online lists like those found on Goodreads (https://www.goodreads.com/).
Expert facilitators	Check colleges for a list of faculty experts and their areas of expertise.
	Consider specialists from related businesses and industries.
	Recruit hobbyists.
	Review the teachers/instructors for relevant K-12 or college courses.
	Use community partners as facilitators.

successful projects. The overall take away is to simply try the model for a few topics and adapt from there. It can provide a low stress replicable design for library collaboration with community partners.

Note

1 Literacy categories reflect the five essential PA Forward literacies (Pennsylvania Library Association, 2018).

References

ALAStore. (n.d.). *Reader's advisory series*. Retrieved from https://www.alastore.ala.org/search-store?search_api_views_fulltext=%22Readers%27+Advisory+Guide%22

American Library Association. (2018). *Let's talk about it*. Retrieved from http://www.ala.org/tools/programming/ltai

Auel, J. L. (2011). *Land of the painted caves.* New York, NY: Crown.

Cobb, H. (2010). *Paths of glory.* New York, NY: Penguin Books.

Hertzog, W. (Director). (2011). *Cave of forgotten dreams* [Motion picture]. United States: MPI Home Video.

Hooper, B. (2016). *The librarian's guide to book programs and author events.* Chicago: ALA Editions, an imprint of the American Library Association.

Irons, K. (2014). *Film programming for public libraries.* Chicago, IL: ALA.

Kubrick, S. (Director). (2006). *Paths of glory* [Motion picture]. United States: MGM.

Larson, E. (2006). *Thunderstruck.* New York, NY: Crown.

Maccaferri, J. (2017). [Promotional materials]. Copies in possession of James T. Maccaferri, Clarion University of Pennsylvania, Clarion, PA.

Moorehead, A. (2002). *Gallipoli.* New York, NY: HarperCollins.

NoveList. (2016). *Cooking the books: Food programs in libraries* [Video file]. Retrieved from https://www.youtube.com/watch?v=xuTyeN8w1R8&t=2s

Office of Public Programming, American Library Association. (2018). *The benefits of public programming for participating libraries and audiences* [web page]. Retrieved from http://www.ala.org/aboutala/offices/ppo/resources/benefitspublic

Pennsylvania Library Association. (2018). *PA Forward.* Retrieved from http://www.pa-forward.org/

Pennsylvania Library Association. (n.d.). What are the five literacies? Retrieved from http://www.paforward.org/Portals/0/Docs/The%20Five%20Literacies.pdf

Pushing the Limits. (2017). *Guide to pushing the limits.* Retrieved from http://pushingthelimits.org/bhome/professional-development-b/unit-1-adult-stem-programs-in-your-library-b/

Pushing the Limits. (n.d.). *Adult STEM programs in your library.* Retrieved from http://pushingthelimits.org/ahome/pd-home/pdunit1/

Robertson, D. A. (2005). *Cultural programming for libraries: Linking libraries, communities, and culture.* Chicago. IL: American Library Association.

Schwartz, M. (2012). *Pushing the limits grants teach science through fiction. Library Journal.* Retrieved from https://lj.libraryjournal.com/2012/10/library-services/pushing-the-limits-grants-teach-science-through-fiction/#_

Tuchman, B. (1994). *The guns of August.* New York, NY: Random House.

Weir, P. (Director). (2017). *Gallipoli* [Motion picture]. United States: Paramount.

Zickuhr, K., Rainie, L. & Purcell, K. (2013). *Library services in the digital age: Part 4: What people want from their libraries.* Retrieved from http:// libraries.pewinternet.org/2013/01/22/part-4-what-people-want-from-their-libraries/

13

THE CARVER CUBS SUMMER BOOK CLUB

A reciprocal collaboration between a neighborhood library and a graduate elementary teacher preparation program

Estanislado S. Barrera IV, Kim Skinner, and Brandon Reilly

This exemplar discusses the development and maintenance of the Carver Cubs Summer Book Club, an academic service-learning partnership between East Baton Rouge Parish Library System's (EBRPLS) Carver Branch Library and the Elementary Holmes Teacher Preparation Program at Louisiana State University (LSU). Through this six-year collaboration, the partnership has provided a multi-week, reading-intensive program which increased children's exposure to literature, positively affected children's reading enjoyment, and improved children's reading abilities and comprehension skills. In the discussion that follows, we provide a description of the project and identify the specific goals associated with the partnership. Our discussion will then shift to give attention to beginning the partnership, how it functions, and the reciprocal nature of the relationship. The illustration will conclude by discussing the outcomes, lessons learned, and recommendations for others interested in similar community partnerships.

The Carver Cubs Book Club

The joint efforts of the partnership yielded the development of The Carver Cubs Summer Book Club. The reciprocal goals of the partnership were (1) providing free instruction and enrichment to the young patrons (elementary age) of the neighborhood library during the summer through small group and individual reading instruction, and (2) creating opportunities for preservice teachers to refine their skills associated with teaching reading and to gain experience working with diverse student populations.

To accomplish the established goals, the book club – which is similar to a reading clinic – met each June for at least 20 one-hour sessions. In keeping with a clinical model, the university students provided specific, individualized reading and writing intervention and small-group instruction based on diagnostic literacy assessment data.

Each session of the Carver Cubs Summer Book Club began with the children arriving and sign-in with the children's librarian. Next, the graduate students serving as their "teachers" greeted the children and escorted them to the particular area/group where they would read and write. Intended to increase motivation and engagement with text, children freely chose not only the particular text they would read and/or use as a mentor text, they also chose all books used for instruction. Each book club session ended with a snack (provided by the library) and a "wrap-up" activity articulating accomplishments and plans for the next day. Afterwards, the preservice teachers walked out with the young patrons and dismissed them to either walk home or be picked up by a parent/caregiver. This was also a great time for the preservice teachers to speak to any parents who were waiting for their child.

At the final meeting of each book club, parents/caregivers were given summary reports for each patron that included reading assessment data, progress made during the sessions, and information that could be shared with teachers. Pizza and juice were sponsored by EBRPLS and reusable bags from a bookstore filled with children's books and school supplies are provided to each participating patron thanks to a grant from the University Presbyterian Church on our campus.

A reciprocal partnership

Zlotkowski's (1999) Conceptual Service-Learning Matrix informed the basis for this project, which emphasized the nexus of community partnership, pedagogical strategies, and reflection. The following section will provide background on each of the partners – Carver Branch Library and the Elementary Holmes Program – and then describe how the partnership began and continues to function in a reciprocal relationship.

Carver Branch Library. One of 13 branches in EBRPLS, the Carver Branch Library is located in Old South Baton Rouge which is the oldest African American neighborhood of Baton Rouge, Louisiana (Hendry & Edwards, 2009). Centrally situated on a main thoroughfare, Carver is surrounded by single-family homes, privately owned businesses, a church, and a grocery store. This library is vital to the community it serves because in addition to the provision of books, audiotapes, and reference materials, the library provides patrons access to computers, internet, email, online applications, printing, copying, and other necessities.

Articulated on the library system website, the mission statement of East Baton Rouge Parish Library (EBRPLS) is "a community service organization that connects our citizens with information, resources, materials, technology, and experiences in order to make a positive difference in their lives" (EBRPLS, n.d., para. 1). Exemplifying EBRPLS's mission, the branch manager identified providing summer programming for the elementary-aged patrons who lived in the neighborhood as his primary focus. Many of these young patrons were home all day during the summer months and would spend their time at the library, but the main attraction for them was access to the computers for web-based games and internet resources. Although the library staff willingly provided this service, computer time was limited due to heavy demand. After 30 minutes of use, patrons had to wait until it was their turn again – this was the only way to provide accessibility to the computers for all patrons. This downtime was what the branch manager at Carver wanted to address.

Through coordinated event scheduling managed by EBRPLS, the branch did have a variety of programs for the young patrons scheduled throughout the summer, but most offerings occurred only one hour once a week. The branch manager and librarians wanted something more consistent, educational, and impactful.

The parents. The parents of the neighborhood were also an important part of the partnership because the parents' support was crucial to the success of the summer reading club. Their appreciation for education and literacy and their trust in the Carver Library is the reason why they gave permission for their child(ren) to participate, ensured their child(ren) had daily transportation, observed interaction between children and preservice teachers, questioned tutors about their children's progress, and participated in final meeting of each two-week book club.

Elementary Holmes Program. The Elementary Holmes Program participated in this project through two graduate reading courses offered every summer. The first course, Teaching Reading in the Elementary School, addresses the knowledge and skill elementary school teachers need for instruction of phonics, fluency, and reading and listening comprehension of narrative text. The second course, Content Area Reading, addresses the knowledge and skill elementary school teachers need for reading comprehension and vocabulary instruction of informational text.

Both Barrera and Skinner, LSU faculty in the School of Education, had previously taught the two courses and felt that an academic service-learning opportunity provided preservice teachers with concrete experiences of working with children in the areas of reading and writing instruction. Additionally, the library setting offered access to children's literature, a necessity for student teachers to understand the differences between and how to teach the numerous genres of text.

The university education students' practicum schedule for each of the 20 sessions was 120 minutes of course content and practice; 30 minutes of planning time with peers; 60 minutes of targeted, child-centered reading and writing instruction; followed by 30 minutes of reflection on previous instruction and the next steps for children. The graduate reading courses' enrollment has averaged 25–30 students for the last six years. Demographically, the participants have been 100% female with 88% self-identified as "white", 8% self-identified as "black", and 4% self-identified as "Hispanic". These preservice teachers are all in their early- to mid-twenties and represent diverse socio-economic backgrounds.

The partnership begins. This partnership began as a result of a networking event hosted by LSU's Center for Community Engagement, Learning, and Leadership (CCELL) which facilitates service-learning courses and community partnerships and provides supports for sustaining the collaborations. At this event that was held towards the end of Spring 2013, the Assistant Director of the East Baton Rouge Parish Library System (EBRPLS) approached CCELL's staff with concerns for some of the library system's young patrons because many of them were school-aged children and visited a particular branch library for an extended time each day during the summer. The Assistant Director believed the children would benefit from a regularly scheduled educational program focused on reading improvement. Being aware of this identified need, CCELL immediately connected the Assistant Director of EBRPLS with the two university faculty members who were also attending the event. The three individuals discussed ways a reading education service-learning course could assist these young library patrons and this initial phase of networking was the beginning of a very successful and ongoing partnership.

The next phase began with LSU's faculty meeting with the Carver branch manager and the children's librarian to evaluate ways for this collaborative partnership to be effective, sustainable, and reciprocal. Over the next month, university and library collaborators were in regular contact with one another by phone and email to ensure that all knew how the book club was evolving, and to share any decisions that required input from stakeholders. In addition to as-needed communication, weekly check-ins and updates occurred to address issues such as changes to event calendars and logistical needs, since the graduate reading courses would also take place at the library (see Table 13.1).

TABLE 13.1 Establishing the reciprocal partnership

Date(s)	Action(s)	Individuals Responsible
May 2013	Attended end-of-year event and network	CCELL, Elementary Holmes, and Carver Library
	Initial partnership meeting with all stakeholders	CCELL, Elementary Holmes, and Carver Library
	Identify the benefits and needs for a reciprocal relationship	Elementary Holmes and Carver Library
	Revise course syllabus to align to partnership's needs	Elementary Holmes
	Begins recruiting patrons	Carver Library
	Final planning and approval meeting	Elementary Holmes and Carver Library
June 2013	Prepare for book club to begin (set-up materials)	Elementary Holmes and Carver Library
	First day for book club	Elementary Holmes and Carver Library

The reciprocal relationship. Since the beginning, the team functioned as a cohesive unit whose "commitment [took] the form of doing strategic planning together [and] intentionally developing interdependent agendas" (Morton, 1995, p. 30). This approach maintained the mutual respect and appreciation that is so critical to any successfully functioning partnership. This involved all members of the partnership offering their skills and expertise (see Figure 13.1). It has also involved everyone actively contributing through sharing the workload.

As with any successful partnership, the roles and functions of those involved were modified and adjusted over the course of the six years that the book club occurred. This was primarily based on staffing and availability of the partners themselves. There were times when both the university faculty members could not be involved due to summer teaching assignments and there were instances when the library staff's schedules could not accommodate the book club's meeting time.

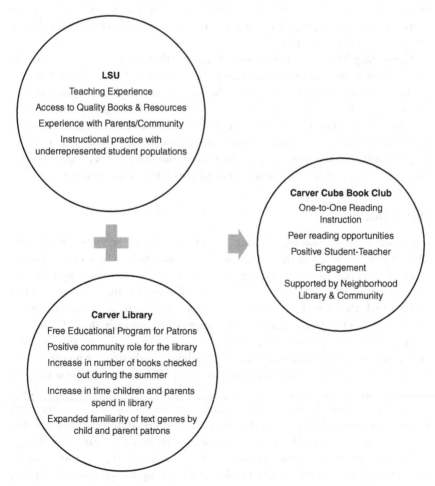

LSU
Teaching Experience
Access to Quality Books & Resources
Experience with Parents/Community
Instructional practice with underrepresented student populations

Carver Cubs Book Club
One-to-One Reading Instruction
Peer reading opportunities
Positive Student-Teacher Engagement
Supported by Neighborhood Library & Community

Carver Library
Free Educational Program for Patrons
Positive community role for the library
Increase in number of books checked out during the summer
Increase in time children and parents spend in library
Expanded familiarity of text genres by child and parent patrons

FIGURE 13.1 Partnership.

However, despite these obstacles, the partnership was capable of handling change because these changes were addressed with ample time to adjust and evolve to demands of the new situation for that particular summer.

Carver Library's contribution. The most significant contribution that Carver Library offered was the opportunity for preservice teachers to engage with elementary-aged developing readers as well as their parents/caregivers. This was accomplished because the children's librarian orchestrated the recruiting and registering of the young patrons and collected parent contact information and signed-permission forms. Because the setting was a library, it also offered considerable access to quality children's literature and other educational materials and programing that were beneficial to achieving the instructional goals of the two graduate courses. With respect to programming, the library put forth effort to schedule events that complemented the book club but did not conflict with instructional time. Allowing the two courses to meet in the library's two large event rooms was yet another benefit. The library provided snacks for the patrons every day and also organized the award ceremony through help from local government programs and grants.

Elementary Holmes contributions. Recalling that the Carver Library's primarily purpose was to provide an engaging service for their youngest patrons, the most significant contribution that the Elementary Holmes program and its graduate students provided was the individualized and small-group instructional time and application of intervention strategies that fostered reading and writing improvement related to comprehension development. In addition to benefitting the children, the preservice teachers also communicated with the parents/caregivers and provided them with data and instructional recommendations.

Outcomes

Important to understanding the success of this academic service-learning collaboration is the role that the participatory approach played "as it highlights the value of reciprocity in developing and maintaining a service-learning relationship" (Tinkler et al., 2014). Over the course of six years, the collaboration has transformed, always with the goal of improvement – for the book club, the reading courses, and the partnership. The Carver Cubs Summer Book Club consistently serves 30–45 children each summer, and requests for attendance have grown beyond the boundaries of the neighborhood – although not honored. The library branch manager indicated that providing this summer program has also caused an increase in the quantity of visits by patrons during the month of June.

The library branch manager also found that this continued partnership was the only initiative that was sustained over time. While different urban renewal grants and projects would appear for a few months or a few years, they always disappeared when the funding ended, or the original investigators moved on to another project. Sometimes individuals would sign up to volunteer their time, not realizing the commitment and understanding required in this community.

TABLE 13.2 Measurable outcomes per year

Summer	Number of University Student Tutors	Number of Young Patrons Served	Number of Hours in Library
2013	28	31	40
2014	17	38	40
2015	29	44	40
2016	17 + 12 (two courses)	47 + 26 (2nd reading camp offered in morning)	50 + 50
2017	23 + 21 (two courses)	46 + 37 (both offered in afternoon)	50 + 50
2018	23 + 24 (two courses)	50 + 41 (both offered in afternoon)	50 + 50

For example, Carver Branch Library is a federal worksite for university work-study students. While students self-select to tutor children and teens after school at the library, some are not prepared for the nature of the job. University students often request to shelve books rather than work with children. This six-year partnership between the library and the elementary teacher preparation program is the longest sustained project in Carver's history. As for the young patrons, they benefited by participating in a free book club that offered specific instruction to improve reading and writing. They also benefit from experiencing their neighborhood library as a community resource and place that cares for them. Participation in the book club also provided the patrons with an opportunity to engage in a positive student-teacher relationship due to the one-to-one instructional format. This particular experience demonstrated to the patrons that their book club teacher cared about them and was interested in helping them. Because this relationship was an academic service-learning partnership, the faculty members were able to secure funding through university sponsored programs to provide the patrons with school supplies and books.

Overall, the outcomes have been the partnership's ability to offer a free summer reading and writing enrichment program that has improved consistently in regard to its ability to serve young developing readers and to prepare preservice teachers for their clinical experiences. The project has also fostered new partnerships between the local library branches and other literacy-focused courses (Table 13.2).

Challenges and lessons learned

As with all endeavors, there were challenges, but the dedication of the partners has helped turn the challenges into lessons learned. One of the biggest lessons we learned was the importance of scheduling with respect to the lives of the children who were participating in the summer camp. Children participated on a voluntary basis and many children were responsible for physically getting to the library by themselves, either walking or riding their bike. Structure often falls away in the summer, and many of the children reported staying up late, thus having a hard time arriving on time the year we started the book club at 9am. Attendance dropped the summer we changed one course to a morning time slot, and the following years we kept both courses in the afternoon so to maximize young people's attendance.

We also implemented a mandatory attendance rule that required parents' assurance and signature on permission forms that their child(ren) would attend each day the book club was offered in the particular two-week session. By dividing the book club sessions into two, two-week sessions, parents could choose to have their children attend one or both sessions, depending on other obligations such as day camps and family trips. In spite of the strict attendance policy for participation each session, most children attended both consecutive two-week sessions. This was primarily because the students were given free books and school supplies on the last day of the book club during an awards ceremony. We also learned to create handwritten invitations for parents and caregivers, so they felt welcome and wanted at the final celebration. As children "aged out" of the elementary-aged target population (5–11 years old), repeaters often returned summer after summer and begged to be included. Although we prioritized servicing those patrons who were the acceptable age, we always allowed the older patrons to participate because they had demonstrated being a dedicated member of the book club over the years and showed effort towards becoming better readers and writers.

Recommendations and implications

Each partnership will have its successes and its challenges, but there are some general recommendations that should be considered. First, the collaboration has to be organic and authentic in order for it to be engaging and impactful. It cannot be a one-sided and preconceived project that is being forced on the other partner. This was accomplished through focusing on providing the young patrons with a quality educational experience and it required that both partners – the university faculty and the library branch – make changes in order to accomplish the goal.

Had either partner taken a one-sided approach, the community service being provided would have been unsuccessful. For example, if the library had been unwilling to adapt its schedule of events and provide the physical space for the graduate courses to meet, then the university partner would have been negatively impacted because instructional time would be lost due to the students needing to travel to the library after going to class at the university campus. Or, what if the university faculty were unwilling to modify the course syllabi and assignments to align to the needs and requirements of providing a successful summer book club? This could have resulted in the graduate students be overburdened with additional responsibilities.

Another recommendation is that everyone involved must be willing to do the work. Community-engagement collaborations are not easy and cannot survive if only one side of the partnership or one individual is carrying the entire load. For example, each member of the library staff always demonstrated a willingness to assist in any way possible during the book club sessions. They not only provided snacks for the patrons but served them and assisted in cleaning up afterwards. The university faculty and graduate students also contributed during snack time if they had completed their lesson for that day.

Finally, the significance of clear and frequent communication was highly stressed enough. One way that this was accomplished was by partners having a check-in prior to each day and a quick debriefing after each session. The check-ins were sometimes conducted while the partners were setting up the room with tables and chairs. The debriefings sometimes occurred while the partners were both helping pass out snacks or cleaning up. What is important is that a means to communicate is established and that everyone feels comfortable sharing ideas and concerns with one another – it is through this practice that challenges become lessons learned and continuous improvements are made.

Conclusion

The longevity of our reciprocal partnership supports Furco's (2000) argument that service-learning partnerships hold the "intention to equally benefit the provider and the recipient of the service as well as to ensure equal focus on both the service being provided and the learning that is occurring" (p. 12). It is through the reciprocal goals of the library/university partnership that reading instruction and enrichment continue to be provided for young library patrons during the summer. Additionally, this collaboration generates opportunities for preservice teachers to refine their skills teaching reading and gaining experience working with diverse student populations.

References

East Baton Rouge Parish Library. (n.d.). Retrieved from https://www.ebrpl.com/aboutus.html

Furco, A. (2000). Service-learning: A balanced approach to experiential education. *Introduction to service-learning toolkit,* (pp. 9–17). Washington, DC: Campus Compact.

Hendry, P. M., & Edwards, J. D. (2009). *Old south Baton Rouge: The roots of hope.* Lafayette: University of Louisiana Press.

Morton, K. (1995). The irony of service: Charity, project, and social change in service-learning. *Michigan Journal of Community Service Learning, 2,* 19–32.

Tinkler, A., Tinkler, B., Gerstl-Pepin, C., & Mugisha, V. M. (2014). The promise of a community-based, participatory approach to service-learning in teacher education. *Journal of Higher Education, Outreach, and Engagement, 18,* 209–232.

Zlotkowski, E. (1999). Pedagogy of engagement. In R. Bringle (Ed.), *Colleges and universities as citizens* (pp. 96–120). Boston, MA: Allyn & Bacon.

14

THE MONTHLY HEALTH TALK

How a consumer health library became a hub for a successful health education event through partnerships and community engagement

Rita Kang, Phyllis Mancini, Valeria Raivich, and Miu Lin Wong

Toronto Western Hospital, Toronto General Hospital, Princess Margaret Cancer Centre, Toronto Rehab Institute, and Michener Institute of Education comprise the University Health Network (UHN) — the Canadian academic health science center affiliated with the University of Toronto. UHN employs approximately 20,000 people, has 1,272 inpatient beds, and services over 100,000 emergency department visits per year (University Health Network, 2018). The Toronto Western Hospital site in particular is proximal to several ethnic communities in the city, including Chinatown, Portuguese Village, Little Italy, and Koreatown.

UHN's Patient Education Program (PEP) works to ensure that health-care providers of UHN have the appropriate tools and competencies to meet the needs of diverse patients, families, and caregivers. As a consumer health library under the PEP, The Paul B. Helliwell Patient & Family Library at Toronto Western Hospital (TWH PFL) supports patient education programming by offering reliable health information through a multilingual print and online collection of brochures (www.uhnpatienteducation.ca), as well as books, videos, e-books, audiobooks, and classes. The TWH PFL services are provided free of charge to its more than 16,000 annual visitors.

Project background

The Monthly Health Talk is a free health education event led by the PEP and TWH PFL, meant to augment existing PEP services. Hosted at the Toronto Western Hospital site, this monthly health presentation is open to patients, families, caregivers, community members, and staff, and aims to improve participants' knowledge and health behaviors. The Monthly Health Talk began in 2005 as a small-scale initiative in response to what had become a marked need in the greater Toronto area for educational programming that could serve those patients and families with limited English proficiency. Today, the initiative has done much to ameliorate language barriers and provides participants from diverse communities with reliable and easy-to-understand health information in a safe and culturally sensitive environment. The Monthly Health Talk focuses chiefly on prevention, safety, wellness, and self-management. Examples of past topics include: Understanding Schizophrenia, Living with Diabetes, Osteoporosis, Arthritis, Back Pain, Healthy Aging, and Coping with Headaches. The support of more than 100 internal partners and external agencies makes the event possible. Internal stakeholders include patients, Volunteers Resources Department, UHN Telehealth Department, Public Affairs and Communications, Security, Interpretation and Translation Services, and interprofessional subject matter experts from numerous clinical programs. External stakeholders, conversely, include community agencies, Ontario Telehealth Network, external clinical speakers, and sponsoring agencies.

In piloting the Monthly Health Talk, the then-Health Promotion Coordinator first consulted a number of clinicians in UHN to determine best practices for organizing and delivering content. The Health Promotion Coordinator also conducted a literature review to help inform the schedule of topics as well as to devise pedagogical strategies and practical delivery methods for presenters. The main tenets of health promotion were examined in relation to the determinants of health and the health concerns of Canadians. Overall, the literature findings helped inform the features of the Monthly Health Talk that continue to outline its purpose and format until the present day.

As an example, The *Ottawa Charter for Health Promotion*, as developed by the World Health Organization (1986) at the First International Conference on Health Promotion on November 21, 1986, defined health promotion in its simplest terms as "the process of enabling people to increase control over, and to improve, their health". The Charter asserted that eliminating barriers and allowing for equal opportunities and resources is integral to any community-centered endeavor, best facilitated by providing "a secure foundation in a supportive environment, access to information, life skills and opportunities for making healthy choices".

The *Report on Citizens' Dialogue on the Future of Health Care in Canada* (Maxwell et al., 2002) also found that many Canadians are not only concerned with the sustainability and costs of the health-care system, but that they also want greater access to materials concerning prevention, education, and wellness programs. Participants in this discussion, structured as 12 day-long sessions across Canada in early 2002, generally held or came to understand that they too have a responsibility for maintaining their health, while some individuals further expressed a desire to be able to impart wellness-related skills to their children. The report found that more information about prevention and education initiatives delivered by health professionals was considered necessary in longitudinal efforts to promote health.

Pursuant to her literature review, the Health Promotion Coordinator also consulted the *Canadian Population Health Initiative: Select Highlights on Public Views of the Determinants of Health* (Canadian Institute for Health Information, 2005). This document, comprised of a summary of findings of a 2003 public opinion survey conducted by the Canadian Institute for Health Information (CIHI), provided insight as to what participants identified as the significant issues facing Canadians. As CIHI observed: "[R]esponses [to the survey] could be broadly grouped into three categories: Disease or illness, health care infrastructure, and lifestyle issues. Among diseases, the most commonly mentioned were cancer, heart and stroke problems, diabetes, and respiratory illnesses" (p. 5). Important health-care infrastructure concerns included health-care accessibility and waiting times. CIHI also reported that participants identified smoking, a lack of exercise, and poor nutrition as powerful lifestyle-related determinants.

Following the literature review, topics, teaching strategies, and delivery methods were set in the pilot phase with interested clinicians. Although first informed by available literature, topics have subsequently been aligned with the priorities and programs of the organization as well as visitor inquiries at the TWH PFL.

Logistics

Monthly Health Talks are scheduled according to the availability of meeting rooms and of UHN speakers (including clinicians and trainees). Promotion for the event depends largely on existing partnerships with intra-hospital departments and a small number of community agencies. Although the event initially targeted small patient groups, it was imperative that the language-specific needs of the audience and community partnerships be considered from inception. Interpretation was thus arranged live with a ratio of one interpreter to every five to seven audience members. However, today the monthly attendance currently averages 60–120 people and interpretation needs have surpassed expectations. To alleviate this pressure, TWH PFL raised more than $60,000 from industry sponsors, which has made it possible to sustain the growing attendance numbers and offset costs associated with the high demand for simultaneous interpretation. A significant advance in this regard was made possible by the purchase of language interpretation headsets, which allows for simultaneous interpretation to a maximum of 50 participants in four languages.

Format of Monthly Health Talk

The execution of a typical Monthly Health Talk is as follows: Audience members are greeted, offered light refreshments, and encouraged to pick up written materials related to the topic from a nearby display table as they enter the auditorium. The library staff curated and reviewed all written material to ensure the reading level is suitable for a general population. Multilingual materials are also available that day. Audience members are invited to determine their own need for interpretation, which is provided in multiple languages and arranged prior to the event at no cost. Those who require interpretation are encouraged to register in advance and arrive 30 minutes before the presentation begins to ensure they receive a headset.

Subsequently, the event follows a discernable format. The first hour of the 90-minute presentation is reserved for the speaker(s) who lecture(s), usually at a podium, and whose talk is accompanied by PowerPoint slides. Speakers for the Monthly Health Talk are interprofessional clinicians from UHN, as well as representatives from community agencies and past UHN patients. The remaining 30 minutes of each session is reserved for an interactive question and answer period between the audience members and speakers. Volunteers provide microphones to audience members who have questions and any questions posed to the speaker by someone using simultaneous interpretation are able to have their question interpreted into English. The presentation is also broadcast live using a telemedicine provider (www.otn.ca) and can be viewed live by anyone who is unable to attend in person. The benefit of the simulcast is that the TWH PFL is able to reach individuals whose limited mobility might preclude their attendance, or those who reside outside the greater Toronto area. Additionally, each Monthly Health Talk is recorded and archived on the Ontario Telehealth Network website for two years, thus offering even wider accessibility.

At the conclusion of each session, audience members are encouraged to fill out a satisfaction survey in their preferred language and provide suggestions for future topics. Presenters also receive a feedback survey through a web-based survey tool link to capture their own experience in planning and presenting the Monthly Health Talk. The results of the audience member satisfaction forms are then compiled and entered into a web-based survey to be shared later with presenters. Evaluation data collected after each Monthly Health Talk has revealed satisfaction rates that range from 4 to 4.8 out of 5 in various categories; notably, what participants identified as their ability to learn and apply new knowledge, the usefulness of written materials, and overall satisfaction.

Project partners roles

The main internal project partners, and how their expertise contributes to the Monthly Health Talk is as follows: The Health Promotion Coordinator provides expertise in health needs assessment, adult education, sponsorship engagement, staff/patient coaching, and health promotion event planning. The Coordinator serves as a project manager, determining topics after reviewing the compiled feedback and engaging sponsors and contacting potential speakers. Once the speakers' participation is confirmed, the Coordinator meets with the speakers to outline the content together. Topics discussed with the speaker include audience needs, plain language guidelines, and how to work with interpreters. The Coordinator also screens and coaches the Patient Partner – that is, a patient who formally participates with UHN staff in working groups, hiring panels, and other strategic planning measures designed to improve quality of care. Patient Partner Speakers share their lived experience and coping strategies to make the content relatable and relevant to the audience. They volunteer their time, create or co-create the presentation slides and content, and deliver the education. Other speakers of the Monthly Health Talk have included UHN physicians, nurses, allied health professionals, and external speakers from community agencies. The speakers are subject matter experts, clinical educators, and patients with lived experience.

The TWH PFL staff are experts in researching and evaluating reliable health information. They prepare relevant health information in different languages for audience members to take home before or after the Monthly Health Talk. The library actively promotes the event through in-person interactions with library patrons and by posting flyers throughout the hospital. Many Monthly Health Talk participants visit the library before and after the event to collect additional health information. All members of the TWH PFL staff play a specific role in the success of the Monthly Health Talk. The PEP manager who strategizes improvements, markets to speakers the benefits of being involved in a targeted educational event, and oversees the quality and safety of the event carries out key strategic and marketing functions. Reporting to the PEP manager is the administrative coordinator who assists with marketing strategies and communication of the event. The administrative coordinator books the venue, registers attendees, distributes marketing materials to community agencies, and prepares the headsets and display tables. The graphic artist designs the marketing materials (i.e. flyers, directional signs, and posters) and generally provides visual design expertise. Working closely with the graphic artist is the plain language specialist who reviews the promotional flyers and presentation slides to ensure content is easy to understand and presented in a patient-friendly format. The use of illustrations and pictures in the slides is carefully considered. As noted by Friedman et al. (2011), studies found that "illustrated materials resulted in greater patient comprehension than non-illustrated material" (p. 16).

The success of the Monthly Health Talk also relies on the work of other supportive internal project partners. These partners include the hospital volunteers who along with the library staff post flyers, meet and greet attendees, and assist with set up and takedown of the Monthly Health Talk. A long-time dedicated volunteer serves as the moderator, introduces the speakers and facilitates the question and answer period. Given the event is open to the public, the occasional presence of hospital Security is necessary to ensure the event is conducted in a safe environment.

Finally, assisting with the language needs of participants is Interpretation & Translation Services who provide professionally trained interpreters to deliver high-quality simultaneous interpretation. UHN Telehealth Department helps set up the webcasting equipment at the presentation venue and assists with troubleshooting any technical issues that may arise. Public Affairs and Communications send a hospital-wide email communication and post details of the event on the public website.

The main external project partners are the community agencies and organizations, including seniors' agencies, community centers, retirement homes, housing support services, and mental health programs use their connections to promote the event. They also bring organized groups to attend the Monthly Health Talk.

The Ontario Telehealth Network are telehealth technology experts who stream the live webcast and archive recordings of the Monthly Health Talks on their website (www.otn.ca). Finally, industry sponsors provide unrestricted grants to support Monthly Health Talk.

Challenges and lessons learned

Since its inception, The Monthly Health Talk has become a successful event with knowledgeable speakers, high attendance and satisfaction rates and accessible information presented in multiple languages. Notable challenges include: ensuring individual audience members limit their inquiries to two questions and not use the event to seek personal health advice; working with partners who can quickly and efficiently rectify technical difficulties as they arise; utilizing interpreters with comparable skill or experience levels to provide a consistent, audible delivery; choosing safe and accessible (barrier-free) venues, including reserved seating for attendees with impaired mobility; and finally, ensuring suitable time is available in advance for preparing patient and clinician speakers and interpreters (see Table 14.1).

Dalcher's (2016) analysis of the role effective teams play in sustaining successful projects provides insight into the long-term sustainability and success of the Monthly Health Talks. He describes high-performance teams as "highly focused groups that continuously achieve high-performance results" (p. 3). In the planning for the Monthly Health Talk, the professional expertise of individuals and the support of community partners are critical. The collaborations involve effective communication and positive relationships inside the team and with partners. To this end, regular debriefs are conducted by TWH PFE and PEP teams to identify opportunities for improvement.

Recommendations and lessons learned

The Monthly Health Talk employs the expertise and experience of library professionals, health-care providers, patient partners, and community organizations to provide an effective method of delivering patient education to a receptive audience. For those interested in engaging in a similar collaborative educational event, providing high-quality health information, the following areas of consideration are recommended: Planning, Partnerships, Sponsorship/Budget, Marketing, Content, Method of Delivery, Barrier-free/Equal Access, Evaluation, and Quality Improvement.

Attention to strong planning before and after each health talk is essential to ensure the efficacy and overall quality of the event. The multiple tasks assigned to designated staff and volunteers with specific roles for implementation of the initiative allow for a well-organized session, something that can be achieved only through dedicated teamwork and collaboration. The Timeline (see Table 14.1) outlines tasks and accountabilities.

TABLE 14.1 Monthly talk session event planning timeline (May 2018)

Timeline	Task(s) to Be Done	Notes/Contact Info	By	Date Completed
One year ahead	• Annual room bookings every December to reserve the auditorium for the new year	**Contact:** Room bookings	Coordinator	—
At least three months before	• Invitation and confirmation of speakers, topic and outline, date, time, and venue • Explain to speakers about our audience, plain language requirement, interpretation • Confirm sponsors, if available		Coordinator	—
Eight weeks before	• Ask clinician to recommend patient speaker • Meet patient and conduct screening • Set up coaching schedule which ranges from four to eight meetings (interview, write story, practice session) • Invite staff to attend practice session to give feedback to patient speaker • Ask patient to fill out consent forms and take their picture for slide deck • Set up contingency plan in case patient is not able to speak at the health talk		Coordinator	—
Six weeks before	• Coordinate webcasting with the Ontario Telemedicine Network (OTN) and UHN Telehealth Unit to set up live and archive webcasting; send out speaker(s) information such as name, title, affiliation, and email address so that OTN can contact speakers to obtain consent to webcast • Contact Audio Visual department to obtain two cordless microphones for Q & A period	**Email:** webcasting@otn.ca **Contact:** UHN Telehealth Unit	Coordinator	—

Timing	Task	Responsible
Five weeks before	• Editing, printing, and translation of event flyer	Coordinator, Graphic Artist, Info Specialist
Four weeks before	• Request presentation slides from speaker(s)	Coordinator
Four weeks before	• Plain language review/editing of all slides Event promotion: a Send MailChimp campaign to PFEP contacts list & fax to community agencies (including mass media, ethnic media) b Post to UHN intranet calendar c Post to UHN internet flyer d Add to Patient & Family Library newsletter e Post (stamp) flyers at the hospital f Do community outreach to agencies and organizations g Send event details to TWH News, via Public Affairs Communications **Contact:** Public Affairs and Communications	— Admin Assistant (a, b, g) Info Specialist (c, d) Librarian (d, e) Graphic Artist (d) Coordinator (e, f)
~ Ongoing ~	• Registration: English & others • Chinese registration	English – Admin Assistant; Chinese – Coordinator / Info Specialist
Two weeks before	Prepare library handouts: • Topic & language-specific info • Allow time for ordering of educational materials **Contact:** Print two copies day of event for Headset station	Librarian Info Specialist
Two weeks before	• Request speaker bio(s); add to moderator notes	Coordinator
One week before	• Submit a request for four to five volunteers and ask them to arrive at the auditorium at (11:30–2:30 / 12–3pm) **Contact:** Volunteer Services	Coordinator
One week before	• Prepare resource list from PPT for attendees	Coordinator
One week before	• Request interpreters • Send draft/final presentation slides to Interpretation and Translation Services • Must have at least five people to get a language request **Contact:** Interpretation and Translation Services Schedule interpreters' time (12:45–2:45pm)	Coordinator
One week before	• Order tables and chairs from Transportation for delivery to the auditorium day of talk, by 11:00am **Contact:** Transportation	Admin Assistant

(Continued)

Timeline	Task(s) to Be Done	Notes/Contact Info	By	Date	Completed
Three to five days before	Prepare PFEP brand materials and handouts: a Evaluation forms (English & language specific) b E-flyer sign-up sheet (English & Chinese) c Flyer (promo for next month) d Speaker name tags e Blue patient education folders f Pencils/pens (box) g Hand sanitizer h Tablecloths (three or four)		Admin Assistant Coordinator (c, d)		
Day before	a Purchase granola bars (one for each participant) b Buy bottled water c Prepare thank you card(s) d Prepare certificate for patient speaker e Purchase $25 gift card for each speaker f Post flyers on directional signs	Use UHN Thank You Card and purchase Indigo gift card from Shoppers Drug Mart	Coordinator Admin Assistant Manager (c)		
Day before	Charge Headsets • See separate instructions for devices • Take display board, table cloth, luggage and event signs from storage room		Admin Assistant, Coordinator / Info Specialist		
On site set-up (**11:00am start**)	a Upload presentation slides at the auditorium b Post directional signs on main floor, second floor, of the hospital c Post event signs d Set up display table		Coordinator (a) Library staff & volunteers		

	Volunteer / staff station assignments:		Coordinator & Staff
Station assignments (**12:00pm**)	a Snack/water distribution		Volunteers (a, c, f)
	b Monitor handouts table (one copy for each participant)		Coordinator / Info Specialist (d, e)
	c Ask clients to complete evaluation forms		
	d Test Headsets to make sure they are working		
	e Give out Headsets		
	f Assign a volunteer to usher patrons to the middle of the row		
	g Assign a volunteer to hand out microphone		
	h Assign a volunteer to collect evaluations		
For interpretation clients	Help clients with Headsets (sign-out, on/off, volume adjustment)	**Volunteers** with appropriate language skills to help	Coordinator / Info Specialist
12:50 – 12:55	Test Headsets with interpreters	Update template (sponsor name, next month topic and information); follow up with Moderator	Coordinator
LIVE at **1:00pm**	Moderate the talk: welcome and introduce speakers		Coordinator
			Moderator
			Manager
Q & A at **2:00pm**	a Remind audience to drop off their questions into the question box or use the cordless microphone	English questions can be read by moderator; other questions to be read by interpreters (using cordless microphone)	Coordinator
	b Facilitate the Q & A period		Moderator (b)
Closing at **2:25pm**	• Closing remarks		Moderator
END at **2:30pm**	• Clean up and tear down		Staff and volunteers
	• Pack up, return items to library & office / storage		

(Continued)

Timeline	Task(s) to Be Done	Notes/Contact Info	By	Date	Completed
Two to three days after	• Event close out: update registration list, clean out suitcase • Sort evaluation forms by language (give to Coordinator) • Order supplies (i.e. headset covers) • Replace and/or charge Headsets batteries • Complete expense reimbursements • Update CCHF spreadsheet with flyer translation and interpretation costs Post the webcast link to www.uhnpatienteducation.ca		Coordinator Admin Assistant Info Specialist		
Two to three weeks after	• Enter evaluation results in SurveyMonkey • Share results with speakers • Send speaker(s) the webcast link, speaker survey and thank them again		Coordinator & trained volunteer		
Two to three weeks after	Write patient story for the Library newsletter		Coordinator		

It is likewise necessary to actively maintain a positive relationship with existing partners and stakeholders while simultaneously creating new ones. To this end, engaging patients, community agencies, and non-traditional medicine practitioners can be useful for enhancing programming via allowing for additional perspectives, as well as for conveying the value of patient education and plain language. One should also be mindful of expanding outreach to generate partnerships with marginalized communities or hard-to-reach populations. For communities with specific educational needs such as indigenous, LGBTQ, cancer, mental health and addiction, and language-specific ethnic groups, strategic partnerships can be formed to develop an educational series that meets the needs of the target audiences.

The ability to secure an appropriate budget or sufficient sponsorship funding is crucial for delivering a high-quality event. A budget ensures marketing and print materials are professional, and refreshments and speaker honorariums can be provided.

Events such as the Monthly Health Talk also function best when they are able to promote the event through multiple marketing platforms to maximize community engagement. This can include use of flyers, email, website, community newspapers and ethno-specific media (TV, newspapers), public libraries, and internal and external partnered communications.

Fundamentally, the success of any health-related event depends on reliable, easy to read and understand information by using credible sources and having presentations reviewed by an education expert to ensure plain language principles are followed. The use of plain language helps to ensure that participants, especially those with limited health literacy, can read, understand and act on the health information. This may include creating panels with interprofessional clinical expertise and the lived experience of patients. A mixed panel allows the content to be relatable and relevant.

Flexible and creative methods of delivery are also key. Beyond the variety these afford on the day of the event, the use of multiple methods of delivery including demonstrations, role play, videos, theatre, and storytelling works well to accommodate various learning styles.

Equal access to the event can be facilitated by translating flyers and evaluation forms and having culturally specific materials available. Providing interpretation for your target audiences (including sign language) is integral to the success of the event, as is ensuring that the venue is accessible. Doing so generally requires that assistance is available to individuals with mobility issues and sound amplifiers are present for the benefit of hard of hearing attendees.

Routinely soliciting feedback and suggestions via evaluation forms (available in multiple languages), speaker surveys, and informal discussions is required to inform future topics, validate learning goals and objectives, and enhance speaker and attendee experience. The ability to share compiled results with team, speakers, sponsors, and other stakeholders also aids with quality control. It is necessary to approach the event with quality improvement in mind. Reviewing the evaluations and debriefing after each event can help to identify planning deficits and suggest avenues for improvement.

Conclusion

This chapter highlights the important features required to develop a barrier-free and culturally sensitive patient education event that incorporates health literacy, community partnerships, and adult learning principles. We encourage communities, especially those with limited resources to develop collaborative health education events such as the Monthly Health Talk. For those who have access to computers and the Internet, view our Monthly Health Talk webcast at your local venue (i.e. public library, senior's residence, wellness or community centers, etc.). The Monthly Health Talk is a successful model that provides quality health information through collaborations, patient engagement, and evaluation.

References

Canadian Institute for Health Information. (2005). Canadian population health initiative: Select highlights on public views of the determinants of health. Retrieved from https://secure.cihi.ca/free_products/CPHI_Public_Views_FINAL_e.pdf

Dalcher, D. (2016). Thinking teams, performing teams and sustaining teams: Beginning the dialogue around working together. *PM World Journal, 5*(8). Retrieved from https://pmworldlibrary.net

Friedman, A. J., Cosby, R., Boyko, S., Hatton-Bauer, J., & Turnbull, G. (2011, March). Effective teaching strategies and methods of delivery for patient education: A systematic review and practice guideline recommendations. *Journal of Cancer Education, 26*(1), 12–21. doi:10.1007/s13187-010-0183-x

Maxwell, J., Jackson, K., & Legowski, B. (2002). *Report on citizens' dialogue on the future of health care in Canada.* Retrieved from http://www.viewpointlearning.com/wp-content/uploads/2011/04/future_healthcare_canada_0602.pdf

University Health Network. (2018). *UHN at a glance.* Retrieved from https://www.uhn.ca/corporate/AboutUHN/Pages/uhn_at_a_glance.aspxWHO/HPR/HEP/95.1

World Health Organization. (1986). The Ottawa charter for health promotion: First international conference on health promotion, Ottawa, 21 November 1986. Retrieved from http://www.who.int/healthpromotion/conferences/previous/ottawa/en/

SECTION C
Health and behavior

15

INTRODUCTION

Vicki Hines-Martin

Since 1948 and the establishment of the World Health Organization, the definition of and influences on health have been as a global priority. The definition of health has changed from being perceived as the absence of disease to a state of complete physical, mental and social wellbeing to more complex views such as a state that allows the individual to adequately cope with all demands of daily life and the equilibrium an individual has attained intra- and interpersonally. Life's demands can be physiological, psychosocial or environmental, and vary across contexts, but in every case unsuccessful responses lead to poor health outcomes. The interventions employed in support and promotion of health can vary according to the definition to which one espouses.

If health is seen as the ability to successfully cope and function within a complex environment and meet the challenges of life, then health promotion cannot be addressed by one profession alone. Promoting the health of individuals and populations is a complex endeavor – dependent upon individuals, families and communities, governmental and social services, health professionals, experts with specialized skills in literacy and information technology and others whose occupations support the improved functioning of the targeted group. In addition, this perspective assumes that health promotion also requires environmental change because it asserts significant influence on one's ability to function and cope. Examining health within its environmental context is a fundamental principle of health as a social justice issue which is focused on the goals of the highest attainable standard of health, education, economic, social and cultural participation. With the lens that health is based on the social determinants within an environment, there must be a special focus on those individuals and groups most marginalized and underserved within their specific environment.

This chapter presents interprofessional collaboration which is focused on the multidimensional aspects of enhancing health and wellness within a community-based setting – the library. Each of the following exemplars has taken a unique approach to collaborating with other professionals as well as involvement in varying degrees of outreach or engagement with populations or communities to enhance their capacity for health or wellbeing. The populations being served reflect groups across the lifespan and each of those groups have benefitted from a collaborative understanding of the unique characteristics and needs based upon that specific environment.

Library professionals who have led these projects used their intimate knowledge of community demographics and their one-on-one experiences with library service consumers to inform the development and implementation of their initiatives including those focused on food insecurity and hunger, sexual health and resources, emotional wellness and early childhood health. Some of the described projects were self-limited due to the targeted outcomes and/or external influences; others are ongoing and have been expanded to include broader collaborations and deep community engagement. In all cases, the initiatives addressed a previously unaddressed health-related need in a safe, familiar and welcoming environment – the library.

The exemplars in this chapter provide real-life illustrations of the critical elements that underlie interprofessional team collaboration with a focus on health. They include presentation of the processes, strategies, infrastructure and lessons learned as challenges were addressed to develop each of these initiatives. Most importantly, each of the critical elements is discussed in relation to their effects on the identified project's development, implementation and outcomes.

16

DOG IN RESIDENCE

An interprofessional wellness program at an academic health sciences library

Gail Y. Hendler and Julia Havey

Introduction

As libraries navigate constantly changing landscapes of reduced physical space and transition from print to electronic collections, librarians look to their community to identify evolving needs to develop and implement user-centered services meant to transform visitors and libraries alike. Modern libraries, increasingly diminished in size, are reinventing themselves to deliver services and programming that retain goals of fostering scholarship, socialization, recreation and community. Librarians have customarily collaborated with external community organizations to deliver an array of traditional services and programs such as job and literacy training, and programming for book groups and author talks that reflect and respond to community needs. Moving this tradition forward, the Loyola University of Chicago health sciences library developed a unique service to help alleviate student stress by collaborating with nursing faculty and Loyola University Medical Center nursing staff on a wellness program incorporating dogs in the library space. From the beginning, our goal was to support student wellbeing with outreach to tomorrow's healthcare professionals that aligned with the University's Catholic, Jesuit values of serving those in need and caring for the whole person. The program, Dogs@HSL (Health Science Library), would help relieve the anxiety and social isolation experienced by medical, nursing, public health and biomedical students of the Stritch School of Medicine, the graduate programs of the Marcella Niehoff School of Nursing and the health sciences Graduate School. As students transition through rigorous and stressful professional programs, the partners imagined an approach that would provide emotional and social support and educate students about the distinct roles of service and therapy dogs in patient care. Along our journey, we formed a new interprofessional service model and fashioned an innovative role for the library that has garnered kudos for supporting student wellness and improving morale in faculty and staff of our busy and diverse campus.

Dogs@HSL

Dogs@HSL has been in the making for over six years. Conceived in response to community needs and personal interests the program aimed to create a service to support student, staff and faculty wellness with retired service dogs owned by Loyola nursing faculty and staff. Loyola is among the 151 medical schools and academic health centers across North America in making student wellness and physician burnout top agenda items. A growing literature in the biomedical and medical education literature over the past decade has reported a higher rate of burnout, anxiety, stress and depression for physicians and physicians-in-training. Studies conducted by Dyrbye et al. (2006), a pioneer in the field of physician wellness, are notable for widely raising awareness of the problem. An early systematic review identified training as the peak time for psychological distress for physicians and found that burnout is more prevalent in physicians than among peers in the United States (Dyrbye et al., 2006). In 2014, a large national survey sent to medical students, residents and early career physicians found that large workloads, increased competition for residency slots and exposure to human suffering and death caused medical students and physicians to experience higher levels of burnout that peers in other professions (Dyrbye et al., 2014).

No single intervention has proven curative; so many medical schools are now tackling the problem on multiple fronts and focus on creating an academic environment that helps students thrive (Krisberg, 2016). As a Jesuit, Catholic institution with a deep social justice mission Loyola prioritizes the wellbeing of students, faculty and staff. The interprofessional collaboration between Loyola health sciences library and nursing was born to support organizational needs and meet institutional strategic goals by bringing animal therapy to campus to reduce stress, anxiety and improve wellbeing.

Animal visitation programming in schools and healthcare settings is a recent phenomenon in the United States. Intermountain Therapy Animals (ITA) is one of the early and best-known pioneers of using animal therapy to support learning. In 1999, ITA formed the Reading Education Assistance Dogs (READ) program to improve children's reading scores in Salt Lake City, Utah. The program boosted the all-participating children's reading scores by two grade levels and brought awareness of the unique benefits of animal therapy in the educational setting (Jalongo et al., 2004). Within the past decade, academic libraries began to transform traditional library service with innovative animal therapy visits in an effort to support student wellbeing. Yale and Harvard's pet therapy programs have lead the way with innovative pet therapy programming that identified the library as a primary resource for help. In 2011, access services librarian at the Lillian Goldman Law Library initiated a service that permitted students to checkout his dog, Monty, for a 30-minute play intervention. Responsive to campus need, the program garnered very positive feedback from the community and generated a buzz among other libraries for how it modeled how to meet the social and emotional needs of stressed-out students (Aiken, 2011). The Harvey Cushing/John Hay Whitney

Medical Library at the Yale School of Medicine was inspired to implement a less formal pet therapy program in 2014. Students lined up for petting sessions with two dogs (both named Finn) that also proved popular among students. The library does not see this experience as trend, but as a basic library service "that is here to stay" (Xu, 2015). Also inspired by the Monty experience, the Harvard's Francis A. Countway Medical Library's pet therapy program offers comfort dog visits for four hours on Fridays. The benefits of bringing the human–animal programming to Countway has resulted reducing student stress, anxiety, increasing happiness and "making the library a more inviting comfortable place to come" (Bernini, 2017).

Loyola's *Dog in Residence* program was born as an interprofessional initiative on September 29, 2012 when the health sciences library director noticed a Loyola University Medical Center informatics nurse and volunteer service dog puppy trainer walking a service dog trainee in the hallway outside the newly opened health sciences library. The connection between nurse and medical librarian was immediate and natural, founded on shared interests, values and goals. From the beginning, the partners knew that the library could support depressed, anxious, stressed-out students with a human–animal connection and contribute to creating an environment for students to thrive. That the dogs were born, bred and trained by Canine Companions for Independence to serve as the "ears, hands, and legs" of the adults with physical disabilities they served meshed perfectly with the work, heart and interests of Loyola's entire health sciences campus (Canine Companions for Independence, 2018). From a practical perspective, using a service dog population provided consistency in terms of general temperament of the dog, basic training in 30 defined commands and good dog manners in a public setting. Over the following year, planning began on the program as library staff worked on fulfilling the University mandated requirements for certification to launch therapy dog interventions in the library.

The first phase of the program, Dogs@HSL, relied on outsourcing interventions to twice-monthly visits from Pawsitive Pet Therapy, a volunteer organization whose mission is "to share registered therapy dogs with individuals in a wide variety of health care and educational settings – bringing comfort, support and encouragement through the unique healing power of the human–animal bond" (PAWSitive Therapy Troupe, 2018).

The partners chose to work with this group as they were already providing pet therapy visits at the adjoined medical center on two inpatient units, pediatrics and rehabilitation. From 2012 to 2013 library staff became familiar with twice-monthly PAWSitive Therapy Troupe visits. The intervention consisted of a 45-minute "meet and greet" in the library where library visitors would be able to pet, play and relax with the dogs.

As registered therapy dogs, the animals are beloved family pets who undergo (with their pet guardians) additional training to provide support and unconditional love to those in need. The training enables the dogs to function reliably in the healthcare setting when offering animal-assisted activities such as entertainment and visits. The typical visit lasts up to 45 minutes and students can visit with up to three to five dogs and their handlers. Often, the dogs will perform tricks and arrive costumed to celebrate holidays and special occasions. The response to this pilot was positive and immediate. Library staff and visitors were enthusiastic about the opportunity to connect with a pet in the library. Students thanked library staff for providing the "dog break" from studies and engaged with pet and pet parent to learn about the dog and the training required for the therapy dog distinction. Many non-library staff and students related how much they missed their own family pet and how they profoundly appreciated the visits. Library faculty and staff also showed great interest in the visits. Some students interacted directly with the dogs, and others formed closer relationships with dog and/or owner. All library staff took pride in providing the service as they recognized and valued the important role the library played in bringing stress relief and increased happiness to our visitors and the increased visibility and good feelings extended to the department because of the initiative.

During the second phase of the program, library faculty and paraprofessionals learned how to work with retired service dogs and in-training service puppies as deliberate interventional tool vs the passive experience with the dogs from the Pawsitive troupe. The training first covered how to communicate with the dogs using command vocabulary, such as "visit," "lap," "retrieve," "hold" and "drop." After learning the commands, the volunteer dog trainer taught staff to issue commands, properly handle a leash, and safely work with dogs in an academic health sciences library setting. The goal was to have library staff members who wanted to participate certified as a therapy team with the dogs they would handle in the program. Certification programs available locally in Illinois included Pet Partners, Rainbow, and Bright & Beautiful. The American Kennel Club offers a national listing online: https://www.akc.org/sports/title-recognition-program/therapy-dog-program/therapy-dog-organizations/ (Certification cost varies by organization and region, but was not prohibitive for the health sciences library.)

During this phase, a visit "station" was identified. The aim was to locate a space that was visible from all areas inside and outside of the library and accessible from the side of the library service desk where visitors routinely go for assistance. In this way, the team would be located to make the experience less disruptive to library visitors that did not want to interact with the dog due to fear, allergies or lack of interest. The pilot phase lasted several months, which allowed staff to develop a relationship with the dog, learn how to walk through hallways in a healthcare setting, how to handle the leash, how to issue commands, and how to detect if the dog was tired or stressed and how to take care of the dog.

During the training phase, as now, the structure was largely informal with the volunteer trainer holding the leash while seated at a designated table within the library with library staff in attendance. During the visit, the volunteer trainer spoke to the students about how service dogs are born, bred and trained to work with patients with non-visual physical disabilities as the students petted and played with the dog. She also educated on the uses and differences of dogs used for therapy, emotional support and service for a disabled population.

As staff became comfortable and knowledgeable about working with the dogs, the partners co-led the visits. To comply with institutional policy, the library director received therapy dog certification during this phase. A certified handler always co-led the visits with library staff. During phase three of the program, Soren, who was raised as a puppy by the nursing partner and who now lived with her in retirement became the designated library *dog in residence*. Soren remained a member of the dog and human interventional team until his retirement in 2017.

The library partner secured administrative and staff support for the program, managed project roles for library staff. Additionally, she worked with campus marketing and communications specialists to advertise the program and disseminate the library created promotional materials to the campus and our affiliate hospital.

Partnership strengths

The original partner Pawsitive Troupe proofed the concept of dogs in the library. The dog visits elicited a warm, welcoming response to the twice-monthly 45-minute sessions. The subsequent Dog-In-Residence program was developed on the success of phase one and the overall all program was named Dogs@HSL to reflect the diversity and richness of the service. Each partner brought unique and complementary skill sets, shared values and a deep commitment to the benefits of human-animal engagement to the collaboration. The library director brought a high level of enthusiasm and a strong background in library programming, administration and community outreach experience to the collaboration. The volunteer trainer's flexibility, expertise as a puppy raiser for Canine Companions for Independence and experience with mentoring others aspiring to become puppy raisers was critical to the program's success. Most importantly, the volunteer trainer's position as nurse/handler taught library staff how to run an intervention and educate students about the role of service dogs in health care, and modeled how healthcare professionals work with librarians to provide care.

Both project leaders share love of animals and values that align with Loyola's Jesuit tradition. The program has successfully reflected their commitment to care for the emotional wellbeing of tomorrow's healthcare professionals and their vision of deepening connections with each other, our students, and the animals who work with us to improve the health of our students and the future care of their patients.

Current program

Dogs@HSL has offered both bi-weekly PAWsitive Pet Therapy Troupe visits on Fridays which are currently on hold due to volunteer shortage during the fall 2018 term, and which is anticipated to resume winter, 2019. Weekly consults with Miso, a six-year old, Golden Retriever/Labrador Retriever mix is the focus of the program and take place on Thursday from noon to 1:00pm at the library service desk. Another member of Loyola's nursing faculty raised Miso as a Canine Companions for Independence service dog and adopted him upon retirement.

During a typical one-hour session, Miso will provide 20 to 45 "consults." Visitors will find Miso staffing the service desk on his doggie bed with Lambchop, his favorite toy with leash held by a library or nursing partner. Students, faculty and staff can often been seen waiting patiently for a turn to interact with him or kneeling down on the floor with Miso holding his paw, playing and taking selfies. Both nursing and medical students study with Miso. During exams, Miso will lie quietly with a student who holds onto the dog with one hand while reading exam prep from a device in the other hand. From 2017 to 2018 the program became so popular that he accompanies the library director to academic year orientations in the Stritch School of Medicine, the graduate programs of the Marcella Niehoff School of Nursing and the Health Sciences Graduate School. A whiteboard poster located at the library entrance announces visit date and time. Information about Dogs@HSL is available on the health sciences library web site where readers can learn program basics and link to external organizations: http://library.luhs.org/hslibrary/events/dogsathsl.html

As beloved members of the library staff, Miso and Soren are listed in the online library staff directory, http://library.luhs.org/hslibrary/about_us/staff_directory.htm

Word-of-mouth and Facebook posts, which garner the highest reach, remain the most powerful advertising on campus and provide the program partners with insights from the student perspective.

Anticipated and unanticipated outcomes

Outcomes and program support have been both expected and surprising. We did not anticipate the broader appeal of the program would have for faculty, staff and resident physicians, or repeated requests for visits to visit academic and clinical departments. Over the past two years, library visits from these groups have increased due to the opportunity to consult with the Dog in Residence. The popularity of Dogs@HSL among students was not surprising, but we remain delighted by the depth of the community's connection to the Dog in Residence, and to Miso in particular. In the library, the new normal is students socializing with each other and discussing with each other, with us and with the dog, how the intervention calms and refreshes them. A recent study from the University of Sheffield's Counseling Service reports statistically significant improvement in stress levels after students were exposed to brief interventions with guide dogs in training (Wood et al., 2018). We anticipated a similar effect from our intervention. Miso's level of engagement, calmly making eye contact with a visitor and gently connecting with his paw softly resting on the visitor's arm or leg caught us by surprise. It is as though Miso understood the level of distress and reached out to comfort in the best way he knows how. The love our students have for this program and this dog is palpable on campus. We have received informal feedback from all sectors of the community thanking the library staff and in comments on the HSL Facebook page where students called for Miso as "faculty of the year. Feedback to posts announcing Miso or surprise puppy visits continue to earn the highest reach and engagement on the library Facebook page http://facebook.com/loyolahsl. Faculty and staff from school departments and from the hospital who would not have otherwise visited the library now come expressly to see Miso after viewing the poster at the library entrance on a simple whiteboard.

Program support from students, faculty and administration has been extremely positive. It has become impossible to walk anywhere on campus with Miso without students, faculty and staff calling for him by name and stopping for a quick visit. Medical and graduate school orientations are now conducted with Miso who receives thunderous applause when he is introduced as a "health care professional" in service to student, faculty and staff wellbeing (Figures 16.1–16.4).

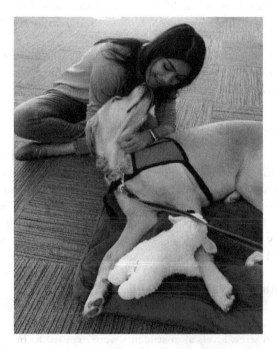

FIGURE 16.1 Miso consulting with Stitch School of Medicine student, Tooba Ghous.

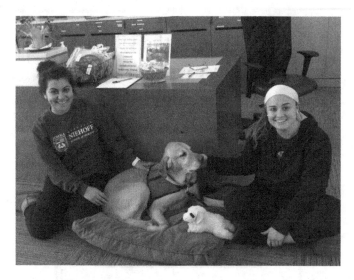

FIGURE 16.2 Marcella Niehoff School of Nursing students Karina Ulanova and Maria Blois.

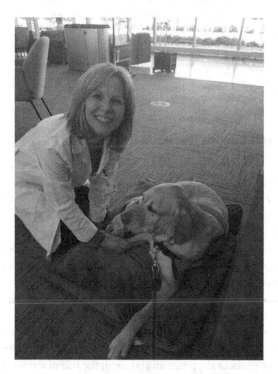

FIGURE 16.3 Burn Shock and Trauma nurse Jeanne Mueller brightening her day with a Miso consult.

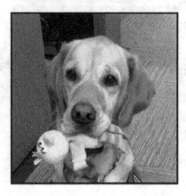

Visit Miso in the Library!

Thursdays at noon

Miso, a six-year-old golden Labrador retriever, helps to raise future service dogs at home with Dr. Fran Vlasses. In his spare time he loves playing catch, cuddling with friends, and socializing with his many girlfriends. Come and meet Miso for a guaranteed smile. He is looking forward to seeing you!

FIGURE 16.4 Visit Miso in the Library.

Challenges and lessons learned

We successfully met the challenges of time commitment for project partners and library staff, certification training and cost, turnover in staff and canine partners, and requests for additional canine consults both inside and outside of the library and scheduled time. The program partners mitigated staff and community issues such as animal allergies and fear, and identified and assigned roles interested staff would eventually play. For staff, the personal connection to the dogs felt as though they were family pets and letting go of them due to retirement or puppy graduation became an opportunity to cement program commitment and experience personal satisfaction and achievement. It is highly recommended to provide all library staff an option to participate in the program. There are many opportunities for paraprofessionals and library faculty to join in that include designing print and online promotional materials, collecting and analyzing visit data, and educating students and other library visitors about the program and about the role of service dogs to patients.

In 2017, nursing and medical students communicated a need for additional visits to support critical junctures on the academic calendar. We scheduled additional visits to accommodate exams, board preparation dates, and around winter holidays, the times guaranteed to evoke anxiety and depression for students, faculty and staff. This year we added "house calls with Miso" to several departments on campus that have requested interventions. Due to high demand, visits to the Health Sciences Division (HSD) administrative floor have become routine after Miso's scheduled consultation hour at the library service desk. HSD administrative staff has communicated their appreciation for Miso's time and have told us that spending a few minutes visiting with him improves their day by elevating their mood and making them feel relaxed, happy and focused. Staff and faculty from Information Technology, Educational Technology, Medical Education, Continuing Education and others have benefitted from taking a brief work break with our Dog in Residence. The good feelings generated by going outside of the library to support colleagues and students has resulted in a recognition of the library as a resource in service to others in a way that had not been previously imagined, but is appreciated and respected. From Miso's perspective, visiting with Loyolans who clearly adore and appreciate him and who stow treats for him in desk drawers is an irresistible benefit for service. There is no cost associated with expanding visits to departments. However, staff time and availability ultimately determine if an additional intervention is scheduled. While we remain unable to accommodate requests for visits to restricted areas on campus, such as the intensive care unit in the medical center hospital and basic sciences labs, we plan to consider alternative options to provide them with animal engagement in the future.

Applications to other libraries

For almost a decade, animal-assisted therapy has gained popularity with libraries to support schools looking to reduce student exam-related stress. Working with specialty organizations already in the community affords libraries a ready-made partnership opportunity to support institutional goals and staff development. Health sciences library staff level of participation will vary. Those who choose to participate will gain a deeper understanding of the importance of the library service mission, and gain an appreciation for the stresses and issues experienced by students from the student's perspective. Additionally, participants experience the satisfaction of contributing to a key initiative recognized by the University making the library a valued focal point on campus. During monthly staff meetings, team members have spoken about the pride felt from witnessing the deep connection students share with the dogs and the deep appreciation expressed to the library for making this service available. Further, by connecting students to each other, and to service and therapy dogs at their point of need, we also forged a connection with students who may not otherwise visit the library. Costs for the program include certification fees, printing costs for promotional materials, antibacterial hand lotion for infection control, pet hair remover brushes and the occasional doggie treats which most library budgets can easily support.

The return on investment is evidenced in increased library staff satisfaction, and subtle transformation that occurs when students interact with dogs and with each other while engaging with dogs in the library.

An increasing number of libraries have reported on the benefits of providing comfort dog visits to stressed-out students in a variety of library settings, but we could find no literature describing an interprofessional team comprised of healthcare professional and librarian providing comfort dog and service dog interventions in an academic health sciences library. We hope this discussion inspires others to be open to new and meaningful roles for their own library by reaching out to potential collaborators in your school to create programming to support and transform the student experience.

Creating the program will take time, patience, commitment and careful planning. Based on our experience, we recommend beginning your process by learning about state laws governing animals on campus and working with Human Resources and the Provost's office to seek institutional approval and learn about your institution's guidelines on animal-assisted therapy on campus. Loyola University of Chicago requires pets on campus to be certified comfort or therapy dogs and display accepted identification while on university grounds. Certification protects both library visitors and the animal providing service or comfort. Animal partners registered as service or comfort dogs have demonstrated reliable and controllable behaviors that enable them to work with a high degree of safety in an academic environment. Certified handlers are trained to detect when the animal is experiencing stress, how to practice infection control with basic hand hygiene, and how to interrelate with animal partners and with visitors from a variety of cultures on a diverse and busy campus. Library staff seeking certification will be required to learn a variety of commands and develop a relationship with the animal to successfully pass the certification. There are costs for certification that vary by agency. The American Kennel Club has an extensive list of certification organizations available online: https://www.akc.org/sports/title-recognition-program/therapy-dog-program/therapy-dog-organizations/.

Scheduling the visits depends on a variety of factors. Let the library's typical busy times, human partner availability, and pet partner availability be your guide. Whenever possible, contain schedule disruptions for consistent service delivery. We recommend communicating changes to the schedule via favored channels with stakeholders to be respectful of stakeholder schedules and to manage disappointment. There have been several Facebook posts announcing Miso leaving / returning from vacation to allow for comments, well wishes and speedy return.

The dog may interact with as many as 40–50 visitors during a single 45–60 minute session. This can be tiring for the dog (and handler) so factor animal partner needs into scheduling. While comfort dogs spend 45 minutes in the library, Miso typically spends an entire day on campus. If planning to have a similar program, there should be consideration for staff time needed to walk, feed, and rest the dog and staff availability for continuity.

Our final recommendation is to communicate... communicate... and communicate some more. Frequent updates informing library staff about changes and program progress fosters greater staff satisfaction and involvement. Solicit feedback from staff and stakeholders to ensure the program meets stakeholder needs. Report on how suggestions were or were not implemented.

Create a catchy name for your program. Write brief, succinct copy about program facts below a compelling photograph that tells the program's story. Assign an interested staff member to become the official program photographer and routinely document the broad appeal and popularity of the program with photos that tell a compelling story of the human-animal partnership. Work with the marketing and communications specialists to obtain permission to post photos on social media. Share the story with the campus, the University and with colleagues. A great success breeds success widely.

Conclusion

Thus far, informal feedback via social media or received in passing from students, faculty and staff has been extremely positive and has encouraged a more formal approach to obtaining qualitative data. Next steps include survey construction to formalize program strengths and identify future needs, and analyzing quantitative data already collected from the past two academic years to determine trends. Plans are underway to meet with campus marketing and communications specialists to discuss featuring Dog in Residence in the University's *Inside Loyola* magazine to gain greater, University-wide attention and recognition.

Interprofessional collaboration based on shared values, goals, interests and unique skill sets combine to create a service that enlarges the role of the library to institutional leaders. Born of a need to improve student wellbeing, the program has deepened connections to our community, to each other and transformed the value of the health sciences library (Table 16.1).

TABLE 16.1 Lessons learned

Program Element	Key Steps	Partner Responsibility	
		Library	Nursing/ Puppy Raiser
Identify program need	• Explore institutional wellness climate and existing campus support • Identify ways in which the program will meet student, faculty and staff need	X	X
Collaborators	• Identify potential partners by shared values, interests and goals • Identify and agree to partner roles and responsibilities	X	X

(Continued)

Program Element	Key Steps	Partner Responsibility	
		Library	Nursing/ Puppy Raiser
Secure institutional support	• Identify institutional policy for therapy and service dogs on campus • Work with Dean's and Provost's office to secure program approval	X	
Goals and objectives	• Establish clear goals and objectives that align with and support the institutional and library mission and strategic plans • Match goals to accreditation requirements	X	X
Training and certification	• Instruct handler on therapy dog handling • Certify dog/handler teams • Identify appropriate age and temperament dogs		X
Program planning	• Identify existing program models in health sciences libraries to identify potential successes and problems	X	
Implementation	• Select time and schedule that works for students, library staff and program partners • Be consistent with visit hours and days • Select a visit space that is respectful to all who visit the library • Track number of visits and record visitor comments	X	X
Promotion	• Create a catchy program name that is easy to remember • Add information about the program and the canine partner under the Library staff directory • Bring the dog to student, faculty and staff orientations and to meetings • Announce visits on social media, library web site, etc. • Go beyond the student population Deliver "house calls" when feasible and appropriate • Work with campus Communications and Marketing to share program details with entire campus	X	

References

Aiken, J. (2011). Who let the dog out? Implementing a successful therapy dog program in an academic law library. Retrieved from https://digitalcommons.law.yale.edu/cgi/viewcontent.cgi?referer=https://www.google.com/&httpsredir=1&article=1008&context=ylss

Bernini, J. (2017). De-stressing with therapy dogs. Retrieved from https://hms.harvard.edu/news/de-stressing-therapy-dogs-0

Canine Companions for Independence. (2018). Who we are. Retrieved from http://www.cci.org/about/who-we-are.html

Dyrbye, L. N., Thomas, M. R., & Shanafelt, T. D. (2006). Systematic review of depression, anxiety, and other indicators of psychological distress among U.S. and Canadian medical students. *Academic Medicine: Journal of the Association of American Medical Colleges, 81*(4), 354–373. doi:81/4/354

Dyrbye, L. N., West, C. P., Satele, D., Boone, S., Tan, L., Sloan, J., & Shanafelt, T. D. (2014). Burnout among U.S. medical students, residents, and early career physicians relative to the general U.S. population. *Academic Medicine: Journal of the Association of American Medical Colleges, 89*(3), 443–451. doi:10.1097/ACM.0000000000000134

Jalongo, M. R., Astorino, T., & Bomboy, N. (2004). Canine visitors: The influence of therapy dogs on young children's learning and well-being in classrooms and hospitals. *Early Childhood Education Journal, 32*(1), 9–16. doi:ECEJ.0000039638.60714.5f

Krisberg, K. (2016). Medical school burnout - reaching out to students at risk. Retrieved from https://www-aamc-org.archer.luhs.org/newsroom/newsreleases/464792/medical_school_burnout_08092016.html

PAWSitive Therapy Troupe. (2018). Retrieved from http://pawsitivetherapy.com/

Wood, E., Ohlsen, S., Thompson, J., Hulin, J., & Knowles, L. (2018). The feasibility of brief dog-assisted therapy on university students stress levels: The PAwS study. *Journal of Mental Health (Abingdon, England), 27*(3), 263–268. doi:10.1080/09638237.2017.1385737

Xu, Q. (2015). Yale's therapy-dog program spreads. Retrieved from https://yaledailynews.com/blog/2015/12/09/yales-therapy-dog-program-spreads/

17

FREE FOOD AT THE LIBRARY

Becoming a point of access for vulnerable families

Elizabeth Lynch and Kelly MacGregor

"Do you have anything to eat?"

Like many libraries in low-income communities, the staff of the Addison Public Library regularly hear this question from children. In 2017, 64.5% of Addison's junior high students were eligible for free or reduced price lunch through the National School Lunch Program (NSLP) (Illinois State Board of Education Free and Reduced Price Meal Eligibility Data, 2017). During the summer, students lose access to these meals and too often find no replacement. Families face many barriers in accessing local pantries, including transportation, few open hours, and distribution limits. Caregivers are confronted with difficult choices between food and other basic necessities. Dropped off in the morning or more often walking with siblings, many children spend their entire day at the library, and before the Free Summer Lunch program, had nothing to eat. Staff kept snacks at their desk, doing what they could to help the kids they saw every day, but it was clear that the problem was much larger than a few granola bars or fruit snacks.

In the winter of 2015, Teen Services Coordinator Elizabeth Lynch and Community Engagement Department Head Kelly MacGregor set out to combat food insecurity in the community by partnering with the Northern Illinois Food Bank (NIFB). Over several years, this vision grew to include partnerships with a wide range of local non-profits and social service agencies. The meal program became an access point and informal learning space, connecting food insecure families to vital resources and information. Lynch first heard about the meal program from a colleague working at a nearby library. She began researching and found that the USDA offers the Summer Food Service Program (SFSP) for students in qualifying areas when school is not in session. In order to participate in the program, the Addison Public Library partnered with the (NIFB) to become an approved SFSP site. The application was successful, and in the first summer (2015), the Addison Public Library served nearly 4,000 lunches.

Staff from multiple departments collaborate to plan and run the program. A large number of staff are required not only to manage the meal service, but also to meet basic requirements of the program. A staff member trained by the NIFB in federal health and safety guidelines is required to supervise each service, so it is essential to have several backups in case of sickness or other staff absences. The library dedicates two staff members – at least one trained, but preferably both trained – to each meal in order to manage the large volume of food and families at each service. In 2018, 18 library staff members were trained by the NIFB at an event hosted by the library and open to other meal sites.

Staff members are also needed to handle delivery and storage. The library is responsible for assuring quantities and quality of the delivery. Each day the delivery arrives a few hours before the meal service and must be stored in a refrigerator. Often, the library has meals or parts of meals leftover from the previous day. Finding adequate refrigerated storage for 125 meals and leftovers is often a challenge. The Addison Public Library already had three large refrigerators and dedicated two entirely to the summer program. In 2018, the library purchased a fourth refrigerator to accommodate growth in the program. For libraries that are not already equipped, the NIFB works with partners to find funding or otherwise support adequate storage.

The Addison Public Library redesigned the Summer Reading programming around the lunch to encourage participation in both. Story times, gaming, STEM programs, and crafts are available to children and families both before and after the meal. Families are encouraged to come early and stay after the meal to participate. Lynch also redesigned the Teen Summer Volunteer program around the meals. Fifty to ninety teens every year receive training, set up, distribute meals, greet patrons, and run literacy activities in the lunch.

Lynch and MacGregor also saw the opportunity to use the lunch as a bridge between vulnerable families and social services agencies. The library uses its relationships with representatives from SNAP, WIC, Northeast DuPage Family and Youth Services, and the local free clinic to develop a schedule of informational tables, program signups, and educational activities. Lynch and MacGregor also worked with the Fire Department, DuPage County Health Department, teachers' association, and the University of Illinois Extension program on special projects in the lunch addressing health topics.

Expanding the program

The program grows every year. At the end of the second summer as an SFSP site (2016) the library expanded the program to include the Child and Adult Care Food Program (CACFP), also offered through the USDA and in partnership with the Northern Illinois Food Bank. The library provides a healthy snack to an average of 99 students every school day and lunch to 125 students on early dismissal days. In the third summer (2017), the library expanded again to include breakfast twice a week. The library served over 5,000 meals, an average of 108 a day.

Because of the success of the library's meal programs, the NIFB invited Addison to participate in a new project combating diabetes. Addison worked with the NIFB, Benedictine University, and the DuPage County Health Department to design a diabetes prevention class for WIC participants. The health department led discussion on healthy food choices, and the food bank provided fresh produce for participants to select after each class. Childcare was provided in an adjacent room, including kid-friendly activities related to the topic in the adult class. Lynch developed an agreement with the food bank to make use of leftover produce, handing it out to teens with after school snacks. Enough was left from the class to support a "shopping" experience for teens, who filled bags with food to take home to their families. This filled an important gap in the federal meals program, which does not allow food to be taken off-site. The second class in the spring of 2018 was opened up to the public, with a significant increase in participation. As word of the fresh produce available with the snack spread, parents began picking up produce along with their children after school.

Outcomes

Although the library's food programs have not eliminated food insecurity in the community, according to the NIFB, they have had a significant impact. The site is the largest in the NIFB's service area, and inspired a growing number of public libraries to join the SFSP program. The library reports over 100 meals a day served to children, but this is an underestimate of the total people receiving food. A "Share Table" allows participants to take advantage of leftover meal components. When a child does not want or cannot finish a part of their meal, they put it on the "Share Table," for anyone to take. In this way, adults accompanying children also receive food and sometimes a complete meal, although they don't officially qualify for the program. The produce taken home after the diabetes prevention classes and offered during after school snacks reaches an even greater number of residents. The students that take home produce are often supporting their parents, siblings, and extended family members. One student filling a bag with apples, grapes, and green beans after school explained that her mother was recovering from surgery and couldn't shop for the family. The fruit and vegetables she took with her would be the only food in the house.

The programs also have an impact by exposing children and families to healthy food options. In our first year of summer meals, one mother explained that the portion sizes in the meals helped her to visualize an appropriate amount of food for her children. She knew that portion size was important, but didn't know what was enough or too much. Seeing that her children were satisfied with the amount of each item provided in the meal made it easier for her to serve them healthy portions at home. The produce available with snacks is often children's first exposure to vegetables like kale or zucchini. Sometimes, even if kids have eaten a food item, they have only seen it in a can or frozen bag. Many could not identify broccoli when it was on the stalk. In a setting with other teens and free to choose what they want, kids eagerly try these new foods, asking questions about how to cook it.

However, access to healthy food is not the only impact of these programs. Food programs draw more families to the library and to using the library more frequently. Caretakers are exposed to the other services available at the library and have taken advantage of ELL, GED, and Citizenship classes, as well as our legal immigration services. Using teen summer volunteers, the library provides programming during lunch, including STEM activities and readers' theater. Teen volunteers read one-on-one with younger children in English, Spanish, and Polish. Complimentary summer programming is available both before and after meals, encouraging participation in literacy, STEM, and social-emotional skills building for children of all ages.

Run almost entirely by teen volunteers, the program also provides meaningful job skills training and empowerment for at-risk youth. Last summer the library trained and mentored 85 teen volunteers. Ninety percent of those surveyed said that after volunteering, "I feel like I can make a difference in my community." The library also supports teen interns, paid, temporary teen staff that help supervise volunteers and provide bilingual activities. The library works with the high-school counseling office and social services to identify students that are on the brink of success, but facing significant barriers. Students must apply to the positions and go through an interview process. The selected interns are given training, mentored throughout the summer, and supported after the internship ends. Students use the internship to apply to college or find their first job. The lunch provides not only structure, but meaningful jobs for these volunteers, who see the impact of their work on the community and develop substantial skills relevant to any environment.

Best practices

The program is successful not because it meets a need in the community, but because it creates a space that is welcoming, empowering, and fun. Focusing on economic need and food insecurity may be necessary to convince board members, staff, or community stakeholders. However, many community members feel embarrassed to come to a program that is for "needy families" or "children who don't have enough food at home." In fact, the program is designed specifically to avoid this stigma. Participants do not have to show need or hardship to receive a lunch. The Addison Public Library uses the word "free," but makes no other reference to economic need in its marketing. Instead, the lunch is presented as a part of the Summer Reading programs already available. Marketing in the newsletter includes the lunch as part of a colorful schedule of weekly programs, encouraging families to spend their day at the library together. Staff also bring activities into the lunch, engaging families in STEM, crafts, and reading. These "fun" activities reduce the stigma that may be associated with the lunch as they demonstrate the libraries commitment to inclusive learning environments for the entire family. Similarly, the library's diabetes prevention partnership was marketed as a wellness program titled, "Get Healthy: A Whole Body Approach."

A knowledge of the ethnic and linguistic identities of the community is equally essential to creating a welcoming program. In Addison, the majority of our program participants come from Spanish-speaking homes where the parents' strongest language is Spanish and the children's strongest language is English. While some of our staff members are bilingual, many are not. Additionally, while some of our staff come from an ethnic or cultural background similar to that of many participants, others do not. In order to bridge this gap we rely heavily on our teen volunteers, all of whom live in the community and understand it in a way our staff usually cannot. Many of these teens speak Spanish at home, and while they are typically more comfortable using English, they are often willing to use their language skills to help Spanish speaking patrons feel welcome. Our volunteers also act as the face of the program, which both empowers them as they give back to their community and empowers the community as they see local teens in leadership roles. As the community becomes increasingly diverse, teens that speak Polish, Hindi, Urdu, Arabic, and other languages present at the lunch are encouraged to use their skills in the same way.

In addition, the library makes adjustments to the structure of the program to make it more relevant to the community. Instead of leaving books out for families to take, volunteers walk around with bilingual picture books, offering to read to families as they eat. Many parents have low levels of literacy even in their strongest language, and in a few cases are not literate at all. Assuming that parents are able to read books to their children can cause feelings of shame. The same is true of the teen volunteers. While a few teens each summer are already able to read picture books out loud in both English and Spanish, the majority cannot. Bilingual staff support those teens by reading through books with them ahead of time, though teens can also opt out of this activity.

Creating a welcoming, culturally competent space can be challenging for staff from all ethnic and linguistic backgrounds. Monolingual staff are often surprised when teens from a Spanish-speaking family struggle to interpret something or refuse to use Spanish at all. They might make comments like, "but don't you speak Spanish at home," that can make a teen feel ashamed. For example, staff at the library asked teens from Spanish-speaking homes to tell patrons at the library about the program. They were surprised to learn that the teens did not know the word "lunch" in Spanish. Bilingual staff, on the other hand, can come across as arrogant or judgmental to teens. They may assume that the grammar and vocabulary they are familiar with constitute the only or best version of the language, dismissing teens who use a different kind of Spanish or judging teens for "Spanglish" constructions. All staff involved in the program must support community members where they are at, providing opportunities for people to learn and grow without feeling ashamed.

The library brings this expertise to its partnership with other organizations that use the lunch as an access point or to reach new community members. A recent survey conducted by the Addison Early Childhood Collaborative found that community members were more familiar with the library than any other

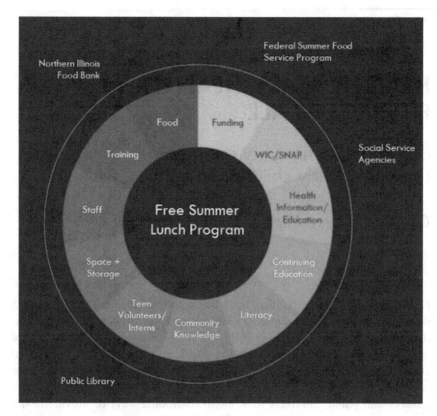

FIGURE 17.1   Free Summer Lunch program.

government agency. These agencies also suffer from community fears surrounding the use of government services or negative stereotypes about their efficiency and effectiveness. By using the space of the library, the same services and agencies are associated with the welcoming and empowering space of the lunch. Lynch and MacGregor work with the organizations to enhance this effect. Sometimes this means developing appropriate activities to engage families, which include people of all ages and literacy levels. It almost always means working with organizations to overcome linguistic barriers. Their information and activities must either be translated or designed to communicate across linguistic divides. The library often includes volunteers in this process, preparing teens with the vocabulary they need to assist families with games or activities. The library provides an invaluable welcoming space for a variety of needs (Figure 17.1).

Reference

Illinois Board of Education (2017). Illinois State Board of Education Free and Reduced Price Meal Eligibility Guidelines Set for the 2017–18 School Year retrieved at https://www.isbe.net/Lists/News/NewsDisplay.aspx?ID=1167

18

HEALTHY START, HEALTHY FUTURE FOR ALL

Building a community coalition to address early childhood health

Ophelia T. Morey, Mary K. Comtois, and Christy Panagakis

Health disparities are a familiar issue for many communities across the US where it is common for community coalitions to be used as a method to address these challenges. Many of these coalitions are grassroots while others are led by organizations such as the United Way who have a strong history of financial and advocacy support for communities in this country. Libraries' roles in these coalitions are not well documented, although it is common for medical/health sciences and public librarians to work in traditional ways to provide health information services in their communities. In this chapter, we will provide example of an effective United Way supported coalition and the librarian's role in that coalition.

The Buffalo, New York area is consistently one of the poorest in the country. Thirty-one percent of the city lives below the poverty line, while the median household income of $33,119 is over $20,000 lower than the national median (U.S. Census Bureau, 2016). In addition to a high concentration of poverty in underserved areas, many of Buffalo's poorest neighborhoods suffer from high infant mortality and low breastfeeding rates. To illustrate, the infant mortality rate in Erie County, where Buffalo is located, is 7.2, compared with the New York State (NYS) rate of 4.7 (N.Y.S. Department of Health, 2017). Similarly, only 18.8% of the Special Supplemental Nutrition Program for Women, Infants and Children (WIC) infants in Erie County breastfeed for at least six months, compared to 39.5% of infants statewide (N.Y.S. Department of Health, 2017). This is significant because the WIC program provides federal grants to state governments, such as NYS for nutritious foods, health-care referrals, and nutrition and breastfeeding education for low-income pregnant, breastfeeding, and non-breastfeeding postpartum women, in addition to caregivers of infants and children up to age five who are at nutritional risk (N.Y.S. Department of Health, 2018b; U.S. Department of Agriculture; Food and Nutrition Service,

2018). The United Way of Buffalo & Erie County (UWBEC) and University at Buffalo MD Physician's Group (UBMD) formed a coalition to address these health issues in their community. The Healthy Start, Healthy Future for All Coalition (HSHFFA) began in 2010, where it was originally known as the Early Childhood Obesity Prevention (ECOP) committee. The first act for this coalition, comprised of physicians and community members, was to reach out to a local nonprofit agency, whose aim was to improve community health. The coalition urged the nonprofit to cultivate a focus within the community on preventing childhood obesity and health equity issues more broadly for children from socioeconomically challenged populations. Initially, the ECOP committee focused mainly on understanding the root causes of early childhood obesity, with the goal of developing preventive strategies.

Since that time, the ECOP committee has evolved to become the HSHFFA coalition, with a partnership of over 40 organizations. Partners in this project include experts from health-care organizations, medical providers, school-based and university organizations, government entities, human service organizations, and faith-based partners. The coalition's primary aim is to strengthen the existing systems and provide community supports that enrich the lives of families while eliminating disparities and improving health outcomes for our most vulnerable populations.

The coalition is led by representatives of two founding organizations: the UWBEC and UBMD. The lead organizations have well-defined and complementary roles, leveraging the strengths of each to form a cohesive leadership team focused on building trust among partners and driving community results. UWBEC provides paid staff, grant proposal development and post award management, community-based research, and report writing. UBMD contributes their knowledge of medicine, health outcomes, and the health-care system, along with making critical program connections from their relationships with medical providers and administrative teams within the system.

As the coalition developed, governance became an increasingly important priority. The creation of priorities and goals helped to ensure that the coalition would achieve its aims (see Figure 18.1). First was the development of a series of strategic priorities: improve system coordination, provide professional development, implement evidence-based and best practice demonstration projects, and influence public policy. Next were a series of goals specific to the coalition itself, which included making the group strong and effective, strengthening the professional field, empowering families, creating policies that promote healthy children and families, and having strong internal and external communications. With a governance structure in place, the coalition then focused on developing priorities that would fit within the primary aim of improving health outcomes for the community's most vulnerable populations. Having a librarian on the coalition for this stage was imperative, because research about the community demographics was needed to ensure that the priority areas aligned with the needs of the community.

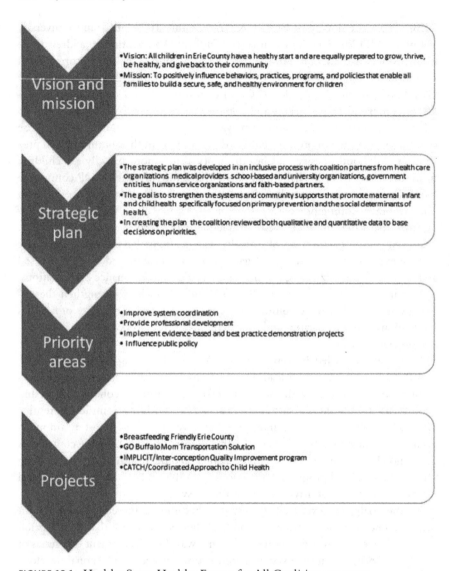

Vision and mission
- Vision: All children in Erie County have a healthy start and are equally prepared to grow, thrive, be healthy, and give back to their community
- Mission: To positively influence behaviors, practices, programs, and policies that enable all families to build a secure, safe, and healthy environment for children

Strategic plan
- The strategic plan was developed in an inclusive process with coalition partners from health care organizations, medical providers, school-based and university organizations, government entities, human service organizations and faith-based partners.
- The goal is to strengthen the systems and community supports that promote maternal, infant and child health specifically focused on primary prevention and the social determinants of health.
- In creating the plan, the coalition reviewed both qualitative and quantitative data to base decisions on priorities.

Priority areas
- Improve system coordination
- Provide professional development
- Implement evidence-based and best practice demonstration projects
- Influence public policy

Projects
- Breastfeeding Friendly Erie County
- GO Buffalo Mom Transportation Solution
- IMPLICIT/Inter-conception Quality Improvement program
- CATCH/Coordinated Approach to Child Health

FIGURE 18.1 Healthy Start, Healthy Future for All Coalition structure.

Having a partnership with a librarian was equally crucial for the next stage of development, where the coalition launched initiatives aimed at addressing the recently determined priority areas. Working with a librarian provided access to research to ensure that the coalition would utilize evidence-based models and programs in service of the priority goals. For example, reducing childhood obesity was determined to be a priority area. During the process of determining a suitable initiative to address childhood obesity, the librarian was able to research existing programs in order to help the coalition narrow their choices down to options which have been shown to produce meaningful outcomes. That research ultimately led the coalition to adopt Coordinated Approach to Child Health (CATCH), a school-based program with demonstrated results in reducing childhood obesity by up to 11%. Another initiative pursued by HSHFFA was early childhood health, specifically the promotion of breastfeeding for at least the first six months of a child's life.

This initiative was enacted through the Breastfeeding Friendly (BFF) Erie County program, where a series of independent interventions across multiple socio-ecological levels were aligned to enhance and strengthen the existing community system of breastfeeding supports. The program first began through a grant from the New York State Department of Health (NYSDOH) awarded from the Centers for Disease Control and Prevention (CDC). The focus of the grant was to improve breastfeeding resources among coalition partners. In addition, this work would link community and health-care services in the pre- and post-natal period through a dedicated staff person responsible to assist in implementing new services and coordinating programming across the continuum of care. Programming focused specifically on populations in Erie County who have low breastfeeding rates because, as reported,

> Erie County ranks 57th among New York's 62 counties, with only 61 percent of infants having ever been breastfed. This is significantly below the federal Health & Human Services' Healthy People 2020 goal of 82 percent. In addition, only 14 percent of Erie County mothers enrolled in the WIC exclusively breastfed their infants at three months of age; well below the Healthy People 2020 goal of 44 percent.
>
> *(N.Y.S. Department of Health, 2012)*

This particular initiative is of importance because the World Health Organization and US Department of Health and Human Services, as well as the American Academy of Pediatrics, American Congress of Obstetricians and Gynecologists, American Academy of Family Physicians, all recommend exclusive breastfeeding during the first six months of life (American Academy of Family Physicians, 2014; American College of Obstetricians Gynecologists, 2007; Eidelman et al., 2012; U.S. Department of Health and Human Services, 2011; World Health Organization, 2017). Children who are breastfed are at lower risk of ear infections, diarrhea, respiratory infections, childhood obesity, and more (Anatolitou, 2012). Breastfeeding has been shown to reduce the risk of infant mortality from complications of premature birth, such as sepsis, and reduces the risk of SIDS for all infants. And, among extremely low birth weight premature infants, those receiving human milk had better neurodevelopmental outcomes and were less likely to have been re-hospitalized after their initial discharge (Patel et al., 2013; Vennemann et al., 2009; Vohr et al., 2006).

The goal of the BFF program is to improve breastfeeding rates by supporting the community of lactation professionals and services through training, improved practices, and expanded support services. To date, program outcomes include the establishment of 29 BFF Medical Practices, eight Baby Cafés (of which five continue to operate), 20 BFF Child Care Centers, 165 BFF Family Day Homes, and 13 BFF Work Sites. In order to lay the foundation to support expanded programming, the coalition sponsored lactation training in which 200 health professionals and community peer supports attained certifications to deliver breastfeeding assistance. This exemplar will focus on one specific baby cafe, Durham's Baby Café (DBC), and its partnership with a University at Buffalo community outreach librarian on the coalition.

DBC is a free, community-based drop-in center for pregnant and breastfeeding mothers which opened in April 2013 as the first baby café in NYS. It is located in a high-need area in Buffalo, where three-quarters of the population identifies as African American (U.S. Census Bureau, 2010) and the median household income is $25,000 (U.S. Census Bureau, 2016). The rationale for a community-based baby café targeting African Americans was supported by the *Surgeon General's Call to Action to Support Breastfeeding* and reports from the CDC, NYSDOH all providing evidence for the need to target and support Black mothers (Morey & Holt, 2015; U.S. Department of Health and Human Services, 2011). Although Baby Cafes have international roots, the DBC maintains a license from Baby Cafe USA that coordinates a national network of breastfeeding drop-in centers to support breastfeeding mothers. As a stipulation of licensure, the baby café is required to have at least two Certified Lactation Counselors (CLCs) or doulas available during operating hours that provide a wide range of services including educating expectant mothers, fathers, and grandparents about the breastfeeding health benefits for mother and newborns. In addition, the baby cafe provides referrals to other community programs or services (Morey & Holt, 2015).

The relationship between the librarian and DBC began at a coalition meeting when the director invited the librarian to a DBC event in December 2013. About six months after this initial visit the librarian began to regularly visit the baby café to learn about the program by engaging with staff and participants. In addition, she also provided donations and helped with baby café set-up, dinner preparation, and cleanup. These efforts to build trust and authentic relationships progressed with the librarian subsequently offering traditional library outreach services, such as providing articles, statistics, information on early literacy, including children's books, and health information resources that evolved into non-traditional services such as grant proposal assistance. The librarian assisted with creating a budget, reviewed project objectives and after the grant was awarded, assisted with quarterly evaluation data reports. Other services provided by the librarian included redesigning the birthing plan to make it easier to read, assisting in promotion of the baby café at community events and via community email lists, participating in fundraising activities and by nominating the director for a community awards. Further, since the librarian worked in a university setting it was convenient to locate faculty and staff who were able to offer the baby café guidance in marketing, including the development of a logo that suggests the importance of fostering early literacy (Morey & Holt, 2015). In addition, the librarian received funding from the National Network of Libraries of Medicine, Middle Atlantic Region (NNLM MAR) to train participants and staff at the baby café on MedlinePlus and LactMed; free online resources produced by US National Library of Medicine (NLM). MedlinePlus is a website with information on health topics, and drugs and supplements while Lactmed is a database with information on chemicals and drugs to which breastfeeding mothers and infants may be exposed. This project also included funds to promote the training sessions and baby café in a community newspaper. Ultimately, partnering with the baby café provided the librarian with an environment to offer community-based health information outreach, and to establish a presence in the community (Dutcher & Hamasu, 2005).

The librarian and director both agree that the lack of funding is a primary challenge to the partnership, for example the librarian has submitted five grant proposals for various projects at the DBC, of which only one was funded. Although this part of collaborating is disappointing, Giescke reminds us that "While the financial aspect of partnerships is important, truly successful partnerships include an understanding of the need to manage the partnership in human terms" (Giesecke, 2012). In addition, the librarian is a tenured faculty member; therefore, time allotment and management were challenges to this collaboration. For example, balancing regular library and community outreach activities, professional development, and faculty status obligations such as committee work, grant writing, conference participation, research and publishing could be difficult. However, the benefits of collaborating outweigh time constraints. In this regard Basler states "success will ultimately be measured in long-term sustainability" (Basler, 2005). Thus, as a community-based baby café, one that is not affiliated with a hospital or WIC office, the DBC has successfully managed to continue operation after exhausting initial grant funds received from the NYSDOH by applying for local grant opportunities, and accepting donations from individuals and faith-based organizations. Community members also volunteer, including the CLCs and doulas who work for free when funds are not available. This demonstrates the collaborative efforts of the DBC founder and director who works diligently to maintain this valued community resource.

Along with the success of this ongoing partnership, comes many lessons learned from which we offer the following recommendations that are also supported in the literature of others (Basler, 2005; Engard, 2011; Gaetz & Lee, 2009; Giesecke, 2012; Johnson, 2011; Stoltz, 2016): First, remember that people may not understand how to best collaborate or understand the partnership process; therefore, the key is to be willing to learn, rethink, and regroup. The focus should be on helping each other to succeed. Second, determine a solid reason for the partnership that meets long-term goals and is important to each entity – discern what is collaborative and what is not. Third, understand that collaboration is not agreeing and agreeing is not collaboration.

> Collaboration consists of inviting into decision-making and into action the ideas and resources of others. It is a matter of understanding the value of a wide range of opinion, talent, and skill to achieve a common good. Agreeing is a mental state while collaboration involves action that gets things done.
>
> *(Gaetz & Lee, 2009)*

Fourth, understanding individual excellence and weaknesses is the foundation to build alliances. Start slowly by partnering on short-term projects as a way to learn about each partner, including you. Fifth, recognize that maintaining independence will undermine the partnership – interdependence is key to successful partnerships; remember it is not about you but about accomplishing your goal or mission. Sixth, invest in the partnership as a sign of commitment; each partner must provide resources, expertise, or other tangible elements. Seventh, develop linkages to foster a smooth working relationship; share information via regular meetings, email, and other communication channels in order to make the alliance work – be open and ready to respond to new information presented. Eighth, foster an alliance beyond the individuals who formed the partnership, so that the partnership may become part of your organization's formal structure – build on present community/institutional structures, leadership, existing strengths, and communication channels. Ninth, do not let financial aspects drive the partnership relationship, remember to focus on the mission and how you can contribute. And last, but not least, utilize a perspective on which to build and maintain a trustworthy and sustainable partnership – trust is key. Convey to others that you are a collaborator by building connections that allow for planning and doing the work. Show that you believe that your partners are competent by giving them authority and by not taking advantage of their deficiencies. And to truly foster trust, acknowledge your partners contributions in public and private.

For those who would like to pursue a similar partnership, one key recommendation is to draw upon evidence-based strategies to inform collaborations. A particularly valuable tool is the *National Action Plan to Improve Health Literacy* (NAP). NAP, first published in May 2010 by the Office of Disease Prevention and Health Promotion, "seeks to engage organizations, professionals, policymakers, communities, individuals, and families in a linked, multi-sector effort to improve health literacy" (U.S. Department of Health and Human Services, 2010). NAP suggests partnerships with librarians by acknowledging the important role they play in sharing information about improving health literacy because they are a reliable source for evidence-based health literacy research (Morey & Holt, 2015; U.S. Department of Health and Human Services, 2010).

Another recommendation is to participate in community trainings. The librarian and director of DBC received training from the Community Health Worker Network of Buffalo, a local organization who works to improve community health using a grassroots approach. This training provided a natural foundation to build a collaborative relationship because community health workers are trusted members of the community who have a close understanding of the communities they serve through shared ethnicity, culture, language, and life experiences where they can effectively promote health in their own communities (Community Health Worker Network of Buffalo, 2011; Morey & Holt, 2015).

Additional recommendations include regular participation in local community, state or regional meetings, conferences, health fairs, and community events (Charbonneau et al., 2007; Duesing, 2002; Dutcher & Hamasu, 2005). This provides an opportunity not only to provide health information, but also to network, build credibility, and identify potential partners with similar goals. This approach also allows for librarians to raise their visibility and increase the chance of receiving invitations to join community coalitions or committees and not-for-profit boards. Further, librarians gain the opportunity to learn about public health concerns or needs and community issues surrounding social determinants of health while strategically positioning themselves to collaborate on projects and advocacy activities to address these issues.

Although developing a strategy can provide a framework for librarians to begin formulating outreach goals for community collaborations and partnerships, ultimately understanding the nature of being in a partnership and how to partner or collaborate is key. For example, the process of forming partnerships has been compared to dating or choosing to enter into a personal relationship (Giesecke, 2012). This process is similar to forming a business partnership where two or more entities combine efforts for mutual benefit where the most successful collaborations are those where partners should begin by putting effort into understanding the makings of an effective and productive partnership (Giesecke, 2012). For many, including librarians, it can be difficult to form a vision for partnering because there are few agreed upon definitions of what it means to collaborate; collaboration is the foundation for building and sustaining a partnership (Giesecke, 2012). The baby café model encourages community collaboration where there are many opportunities for librarians to work not only with local community-based cafes, but with those located in hospitals and WIC Centers throughout the US. In addition, there are baby cafes throughout the UK, where baby cafés began, and if a baby café is not available in your location there are still opportunities for librarians to get involved in breastfeeding or health information/literacy outreach, for example with schools, community centers, public libraries, and faith-based organizations.

After eight years, the HSHFFA coalition is persistent in its efforts to reduce childhood obesity and improve breastfeeding rates by its most recent efforts to support the opening of a baby café in a local WIC office. In addition, the director of the DBC recently received an invitation to join the New York State Governor's Taskforce on Maternal Mortality and Disparate Racial Outcomes where she has invited the librarian to support her in this role. The aim of the taskforce is

...to review and better address maternal death and morbidity with a focus on racial disparities, expanding community outreach, and taking new actions to increase access to prenatal and perinatal care, including establishing a pilot expansion of Medicaid coverage for doulas.

(N.Y.S. Department of Health, 2018a)

While this initiative is in its early stages, it is anticipated that librarians will provide health information and participate in outreach activities. These continued efforts to address health disparities convey the impact of strategic community-based partnerships, such as coalitions, and the value of a librarian who is immersed in these efforts (Dutcher & Hamasu, 2005; Morey & Holt, 2015).

Acknowledgment

The authors would like to acknowledge the Rev. Diann Holt, director of Durham's Baby Cafe for her vision, leadership, and support.

References

American Academy of Family Physicians. (2014). Breastfeeding, family physicians supporting (Position Paper). Retrieved from http://www.aafp.org/about/policies/all/breastfeeding-support.html

American College of Obstetricians Gynecologists, Committee on Health Care for Underserved Women. (2007). ACOG Committee Opinion No. 361: Breastfeeding: maternal and infant aspects. *Obstetrics & Gynecology, 109*(2 Pt 1), 479–480.

Anatolitou, F. (2012). Human milk benefits and breastfeeding. *Journal of Pediatric and Neonatal Individualized Medicine, 1*(1), 11–18. doi:10.7363/010113.

Basler, T. G. (2005). Community outreach partnerships. *Reference Services Review, 33*(1), 31–37. doi:10.1108/00907320410519441.

Charbonneau, D. H., Marks, E. B., Healy, A. M., & Croatt-Moore, C. F. (2007). Collaboration addresses information and education needs of an urban public health workforce. *Journal of the Medical Library Association, 95*(3), 352–354. doi:10.3163/1536-5050.95.3.352.

Community Health Worker Network of Buffalo. (2011). *Community health worker core competencies training.* Buffalo, NY: Community Health Worker Network of Buffalo.

Duesing, A. (2002). Community connections in off-campus outreach services. *Journal of Library Administration, 37*(1–2), 269–278. doi:10.1300/J111v37n01_22

Dutcher, G. A., & Hamasu, C. (2005). Community-based organizations' perspective on health information outreach: A panel discussion. *Journal of the Medical Library Association, 93*(4 Suppl), S35–S42. Retrieved from https://www.ncbi.nlm.nih.gov/pmc/articles/PMC1255751/

Eidelman, A. I., Schanler, R. J., Johnston, M., Landers, S., Noble, L., Szucs, K., ... Breastfeeding, S. (2012). Breastfeeding and the use of human milk. *Pediatrics, 129*(3), E827–E841. doi:10.1542/peds.2011–3552

Engard, N. C. (2011). Collaborative leadership. *Collaborative Librarianship, 3*(3), 174–175.

Gaetz, I., & Lee, J. (2009). Collaboration: The big picture. *Collaborative Librarianship, 1*(3), 99–105.

Giesecke, J. (2012). The value of partnerships: Building new partnerships for success. *Journal of Library Administration, 52*(1), 36–52.

Johnson, W. (2011). Collaboration is risky. Now, get on with it. Retrieved from https://hbr.org/2011/06/collaboration-is-risky-now-get

Morey, O. T., & Holt, D. (2015). *Reimaging community outreach: A librarian in grandma's kitchen.* Paper presented at the Culture Keepers IX: Meet at the Gateway: Reimagining Communities, Technologies, and Libraries, St. Louis, MO.

N.Y.S. Department of Health. (2012). Helping mothers and babies stay healthy state department of health awards Erie County $507,604 to promote breastfeeding. Retrieved from https://www.health.ny.gov/press/releases/2012/2012-12-20_erie_county_award.htm

N.Y.S. Department of Health. (2017). Maternal and infant health indicators. *New York State Community Health Indicator Reports.* Retrieved from https://www.health.ny.gov/statistics/chac/indicators/mih.htm

N.Y.S. Department of Health. (2018a). Governor Cuomo announces comprehensive initiative to target maternal mortality and reduce racial disparities in outcomes. Retrieved from https://www.governor.ny.gov/news/governor-cuomo-announces-comprehensive-initiative-target-maternal-mortality-and-reduce-racial

N.Y.S. Department of Health. (2018b). WIC program. Retrieved from https://www.health.ny.gov/prevention/nutrition/wic/index.htm

Patel, A. L., Johnson, T. J., Engstrom, J. L., Fogg, L. F., Jegier, B. J., Bigger, H. R., & Meier, P. P. (2013). Impact of early human milk on sepsis and health-care costs in very low birth weight infants. *Journal of Perinatology, 33*(7), 514–519. doi:10.1038/jp.2013.2

Stoltz, D. (2016). *Inspired collaboration: Ideas for discovering and applying your potential.* Chicago, IL: ALA Editions, an imprint of the American Library Association.

U.S. Census Bureau. (2010). Table QT-P3: Race and Hispanic or Latino: 2010: 2010 Census Summary File 1. *American Factfinder.* Retrieved from http://factfinder.census.gov/

U.S. Census Bureau. (2016). Selected economic characteristics, 2012–2016 American Community Survey 5-year estimates. Retrieved from https://www.census.gov/programs-surveys/acs/

U.S. Department of Agriculture; Food and Nutrition Service. (2018). Women, Infants and Children (WIC). Retrieved from https://www.fns.usda.gov/wic/about-wic

U.S. Department of Health and Human Services. (2010). *National action plan to improve health literacy.* Retrieved from http://health.gov/communication/hlactionplan/pdf/Health_Literacy_Action_Plan.pdf

U.S. Department of Health and Human Services. (2011). *The Surgeon General's Call to Action to Support Breastfeeding.* Retrieved from http://www.surgeongeneral.gov/library/calls/breastfeeding/calltoactiontosupportbreastfeeding.pdf

Vennemann, M. M., Bajanowski, T., Brinkmann, B., Jorch, G., Yucesan, K., Sauerland, C., ... GeSID Study Group. (2009). Does breastfeeding reduce the risk of sudden infant death syndrome? *Pediatrics, 123*(3), e406–e410. doi:10.1542/peds.2008-2145

Vohr, B. R., Poindexter B. B., Dusick A. M., McKinle, L. T., Wright L. L., Langer J. C., ... NICHD Neonatal Research Network. (2006). Beneficial effects of breast milk in the neonatal intensive care unit on the developmental outcome of extremely low birth weight infants at 18 months of age. *Pediatrics, 118*(1), e115–e123. doi:10.1542/peds.2005-2382

World Health Organization. (2017). Guideline: Protecting, promoting and supporting breastfeeding in facilities providing maternity and newborn services. Retrieved from http://www.who.int/nutrition/publications/guidelines/breastfeeding-facilities-maternity-newborn/en/

19

TEAM VITTLES

A made-from-scratch approach to tackling childhood hunger in Ohio

*Shane Hoffman, Janet Ingraham-Dwyer,
JoLynn Wheatley, and Sarah Schaff*

In Ohio, hunger is a serious issue. Around half a million children in the state depend on their schools for free and reduced priced meals (Ohio Department of Education, Office for Child Nutrition, 2017). These breakfast and lunch programs provide reliable access to a warm, nutritious meal and without them, many children go hungry. The question of food security and the issue of hunger remains during the summer months – what happens to these same children when school is not in session? Currently, only one in ten of these children participates in a summer food program (Children's Hunger Alliance, 2014).

The federal government provides funds that are earmarked to help bridge this summer gap in the form of the *Summer Food Service Program*, known widely as *SFSP*. This program reimburses non-profit organizations, such as churches, community centers, and libraries that provide summer meals and snacks to children in areas where there is a demonstrated need. In other words, the federal government provides funds, in the form of SFSP reimbursements, to areas that need free and reduced priced lunches in order to support this form of food security during the summer months. The way in which this program is administered differs in each state and in Ohio, it is run through the Department of Education with support from several non-profit agencies including the State Library of Ohio.

Organizations that host a SFSP site do not necessarily have to cook the food, pay the bills, or fill out the paperwork. Sponsoring organizations, known simply as "sponsors," are often available to handle the necessary paperwork and allow these community sites to focus on providing meals to children. The sites themselves take on the responsibility to make sure food safety rules are followed and to take attendance at the summer meals, in a similar fashion to what one might see during a typical summer reading program at your local library (USDA, Food and Nutrition Service, 2018).

Once viewed through this lens, it becomes apparent that libraries are uniquely situated in their communities to play a role in the summer hunger solution. During the summer months, activity in the local public library is at its highest point during the year, as Summer Reading Programs begin to alleviate the "summer slide" experienced by students out of school. Without the benefit of consistent teaching and learning, many children see their skill sets diminish during the summer months and "slide" back to a lower learning level by the time the school year resumes. The lack of consistent access to nutritious meals during these months only serves to exacerbate the "slide." Libraries are well positioned to address both issues.

Library programs, including these important Summer Reading Programs, are open to all members of the community, are typically free, and are very well attended. This creates a culture and an environment without class barriers or other stigma; one in which SFSP can be offered easily, freely, and openly at the library as part of its regular summer programming. This unique set of circumstances offers a great opportunity for libraries to take part in SFSP, and Team Vittles seeks to encourage more libraries to participate and fill the summer gap.

Team Vittles is a group of volunteers who happen to work in public, academic, and special libraries and are dedicated to issues of food security and childhood hunger. The group was initiated in 2017 as part of a library leadership institute called "ILEAD USA: Ohio," which focuses on developing the next generation of leaders in libraries. The team saw the natural tie between libraries, summer programming, and SFSP. They sought to synthesize these ties using the leadership institute as a helpful structure to launch the team, build a web presence, and develop an effective approach to advocacy.

The work of Team Vittles, focused on connecting libraries and community organizations involved in SFSP, has continued through 2018 and into 2019 with the support of OHIONET, a library consortium headquartered in Central Ohio. As one of the inaugural Community Collaboration Teams, Team Vittles participated in workshops and led presentations to help clarify the SFSP organization and registration process, connect libraries to sponsoring agencies, and does anything and everything possible to keep the flow of free lunches available during the summer.

Ohio currently has the second largest number of public libraries within a single state involved in SFSP, surpassed only by the public libraries of the State of California. Considering the need and the size of the State of Ohio, complementing existing programs involved with food service will have the greatest impact. In order to support this work, Team Vittles demystifies the SFSP process within the Ohio library community, serving as a connector that brings areas of need into contact with service providers and non-profits who are interested in supporting these initiatives. The demystification process can be synopsized with the team's lead-in at most presentations, "We will do everything possible to make sure that you don't have to cook the food, pay the bills or do the paperwork." This sentence gets directly at the root of the most common objections.

As with many new organizations, the first year of Team Vittles' existence was a learning adventure. As the group examined avenues for creating and supporting SFSP sites, two paths for advocacy emerged. The first path of traditional advocacy involves raising awareness of SFSP among Ohio libraries and supporting efforts to implement new sites around the state. The second path involves working with libraries that cannot host their own SFSP site but hope to support a summer meal program in their community. This second path has relied more heavily on leveraging the library's contacts in the community to create appropriate partnerships.

The first path that of traditional advocacy includes speaking engagements, meetings with key stakeholders, and presentations at professional conferences. The team has presented at local, state, and national conferences and has held online webinars focused on ensuring that libraries interested in the SFSP know that participation is not a task they must handle alone. This has increased the visibility of these hunger-related issues as well as the interest in finding a solution within the State of Ohio. Through this traditional outreach, Team Vittles encouraged and supported the creation of a new SFSP site at the London Public Library, created a referral service that allows new sites to connect with experienced providers, and fielded a number of questions regarding the ins and outs of SFSP. The team has discovered the greatest support factor that can be offered in these discussions is a simple helping hand.

The second path, that of grassroots activism, focused heavily on connecting libraries and interested community organizations with each other and supporting their work in the SFSP arena. Through discussions with libraries around the state, the team found that many libraries encountered barriers to participation that could not be circumvented – some as simple as a lack of refrigeration or space considerations within library buildings. In these cases, the members of Team Vittles share their experience networking with other community organizations to facilitate SFSP sites within the immediate area and encourage libraries to bring their Summer Reading Program materials to these sites as a form of library outreach.

Building on these two successful paths, the team created its first plan, which was brilliant in its naiveté. Team Vittles set out to use the SFSP data and tools from the USDA's website in order to identify areas of significant need without active SFSP sites. Once identified, the group felt it would be a simple matter of knocking on doors, partnering with libraries, and finding non-profit organizations in these neighborhoods willing to host these pre-cooked, delivered, and paid-for meals.

From that point of naiveté, Team Vittles learned that there was a great deal left to learn. This team's collective experience with food banks and creating SFSP sites in libraries did not adequately prepare them for realities of grassroots efforts in the community at large. Realizing this, the team performed several informal, internal analyses and clearly saw a need for a plan to actively recruit community participation beyond the idea of "if you build it, they will come."

The team decided that two actions were necessary in order to be successful. The first was a plan to map out resources already available in needy communities. The available data gave Team Vittles a very high-level view of hunger and food security issues within an area, based upon the applications for free and reduced price lunches in the neighborhood school district. This data also gave the team insight into whether or not SFSP was already active in the community. This same data, however, did not display other organizations at work in the community and did not address the problem of some poverty numbers being under-represented. With this in mind, the team set out to partner with community organizations and to learn as much as possible about the realities of food insecurity issues, at the local level.

Early in the organization of Team Vittles, one Plain City Public Library team member experienced a moment of truth for the team. He attended a task force meeting of the Madison County Board of Health Services in the summer of 2017, as Team Vittles was beginning to solidify its own organization. The Board was creating a Community Health Improvement Plan, also known as CHIP, to address the needs of this rural county which is located to the west of the State Capitol in Columbus.

This involvement in the CHIP gave Team Vittles a well-timed opportunity to test their ideas and to see if library involvement could provide a crucial part of this puzzle in Madison County. The offer was quickly accepted, and Team Vittles was chosen to spearhead an arm of the plan focused on combating childhood food insecurity, with the intention of using local libraries as entry points in the community (Madison County Public Health, 2017). At this point, Team Vittles needed to establish a plan of action to fully implement these support services.

As a group, the team decided early on to avoid duplicating the efforts of other organizations. Being made up of librarians, the group began to research food security efforts and found a very sound plan for engaging the community published by the "No Kid Hungry" organization. Aside from the planning steps, the "No Kid Hungry" plan asserts the importance of engaging community leaders alongside traditional partners in a summer food service plan. While it is a positive step forward to have a site set up that will provide children with healthy meals, it is imperative to have respected and connected members of the community supporting these efforts. The second most important thing the team learned from these recommendations was housed in a simple question: "Who knows what is happening with children and families in the community?"

With this perspective, Team Vittles began to look for local leaders in Madison County with a firm understanding of community needs. This search led to an organization called Daily Needs Assistance, known simply as DNA. DNA is a community center located in Plain City, Ohio, that provides for many needs in the community, including and expanding beyond summer meals. Modeling the idea of community connections, the Director of DNA, Tamara Reed, was a great source of inspiration and information for the team. At that point, Team Vittles was a new organization learning how to connect and expand existing resources as the group created a blueprint for action. The Director of DNA provided the team with copious amounts of good advice and contacts for organizations in the surrounding area.

Due to the connections made through DNA, the team has been able to work with faith-based groups that provide supplemental nutrition on the weekends, county-based groups involved in discussing community issues that range from nutrition to mental health and child welfare, local pastoral associations, food banks, individual churches, and more. Team Vittles has experienced a great response in the non-profit sector as these organizations see the need and hope to support these issues in their communities.

Circling back to the question of "Who knows what is happening with children and families in the community?" the Director of DNA directed the team to the Jonathan Alder Community Support Coalition, known simply as "The Coalition" in the Madison County area, and the Jonathan Alder Schools social worker. "The Coalition" is a meeting hosted by the Jonathan Alder Local School District and consists of the Superintendent of Schools, members of the police and fire departments, representatives of the local Ministerial Association, DNA, and several other groups and individuals who attend this group in order to maintain awareness of current issues in the community. With this knowledge, members of The Coalition work together to ensure students have the best opportunities for success both inside and outside the classroom.

The key piece in this partnership has been the team's introduction to the school district's social worker. This introduction changed the way in which Team Vittles approaches communities and the way in which the team supports SFSP, libraries, and related organizations. Team Vittles begins to pave the way with contacts at the local library, but one of the first suggestions the team makes to libraries is to connect with their local school district and in particular, the social worker on staff. The team has found that these school district social workers are so important that one of the team members leads a side project that compiles contact information for various groups, including school-based social workers, for each county in Ohio.

To more clearly explain the benefits of local perspectives from social workers, and to show how they complement the team's high-level overview, we defer to the social worker's words as illustration:

> When I was approached by a member of Team Vittles... about how they could help to address the food insecurity in the Jonathan Alder Local School District over the summer months, I immediately began thinking about how we could form a team to discuss this in further detail. In collaboration with Team Vittles, we had a team come together to figure out how we could provide a Summer Food Service Program within the school district. We all knew the need was there based on our district Free & Reduced Lunch Percentage (20.89% for the 2017/18 school year). We just needed to figure out where the highest need was and where the SFSP could be held.

During the school year, we have two different organizations that provide supplemental food (weekly food bags) to 136 students. Based on where many of the students lived that were receiving the supplemental food and the F & R lunches, the team connected with the Baptist Church in Plumwood, Ohio. Team Vittles connected with another resource, the Madison County Vineyard, to help begin the SFSP at the Plumwood Baptist Church for the summer of 2018. This program was a success and we look forward to another SFSP in 2019.

Members of Team Vittles have been attending the Jonathan Alder Community Support Coalition on a regular basis to connect with community agencies and to keep updated on what is going on in the school district and the community. We are working together to explore other possible sites within the school district besides the Plumwood Baptist Church for another SFSP. It's been a great collaboration to have the local Librarians learn about all the resources and for them to also help us address food insecurity to ensure the students in our district do not go hungry over the summertime.

This collaboration yielded not only SFSP in Plumwood, but the creation of a food insecurity sub-group of The Coalition as well as leads for possible sites in future years.

This particular experience clearly demonstrated that libraries can act not only as sources of community, but agents of change and action in their communities. Madison County, a county already evolved in the areas Team Vittles hoped to support, were able to teach and reinforce several important lessons. A local perspective is very important to coalition building and as seen in the work of The Coalition, an approach that seeks to support the whole child and includes supports from all sectors of county social services will produce the greatest momentum. This "whole child + whole community" approach has great potential, and when speaking at conferences, the team encourages libraries to seek out similar groups and key players in the same manner. Librarians in communities without this kind of group may bring together stakeholders in their school district, generally the superintendent and school social worker or draw other interested members of the community to a meeting designed to launch a similar initiative.

Over the course of the last few years, libraries have been taking more active roles in their communities. At local, state, and national conferences, one sees presentations on these changing roles, on the subject of community librarians, and on embedded librarianship. That evolution is taking libraries to the point of being active agents of change. While Team Vittles did not set out to do more than create partnerships designed to produce summer meals and educational programming for children, there has been somewhat of a butterfly effect in this process. Connecting the dots and engaging with colleagues at various conferences, local meetings, and regional events has furthered the team's reach and dedication along the way.

These kinds of partnerships, as hinted at earlier, can have additional, practical implications in communities, beyond making summer food available to children. The organizations involved in these fields of endeavor often find themselves similarly underfunded, understaffed, and overworked. When a library or other group comes along and engages the community anew in conversation, good things can happen.

Be the change you want to see to see in the world.

Mahatma Gandhi

The intentions of Team Vittles when getting involved in the Madison County community Health Improvement Plan (CHIP) were simple at first. The group intended to create two new SFSP sites in the county within the first year, track the number of meals served at new and existing sites within the county, and share the results. Team Vittles anticipated a three-year involvement with this plan, at a minimum. The statistics gathered as part of the Madison County CHIP programs could then be correlated with other statistics tracked by the County Board of Health to measure outcomes of CHIP programs, overall. What Team Vittles learned through this process, though, was that additional and unexpected outcomes may be more beneficial.

The team quickly saw the advantages in connecting the dots among organizations, capacity, and funding structures and were introduced to the community building concept known as "feeding the whole child." This theory supports the premise that the needs of children extend far beyond the simple need of meals and food. Partner agencies around Madison County, including the DNA organization and the Madison County Vineyard Church, two organizations deeply involved in food security initiatives, reiterated this idea time and time again.

In order to truly "nourish" the whole child, their needs for intellectual, emotional, and spiritual growth must all be met. Organizations may do this by providing inspiring and educational programming along with lunch or snacks. At some sites that espouse these ideas, children are able to take home clothes, toys, or other items from the "kid's closet." Some sites develop curricula to teach kids to think outside themselves and to dream. These approaches may sound simple, but if one's life is spent wondering where the next meal is coming from or timing your bed time before the hunger becomes unbearable, it can be a difficult concept. This kind of programming can also be difficult for a library, especially a small one, to accomplish on its own.

With this in mind, Team Vittles has adapted our initial goals to include the design of blueprints for less well-developed areas, with the ideas of coalition building and feeding the whole child and fundamental theories supporting these plans. It is the sincere hope of the team to be able to replicate or adapt what exists in the Jonathan Alder Local School District to the rest of Madison County and other locations when needed. To meet those expansion goals, the team will be working closely with the Madison County Vineyard Church, who has already identified areas that overlap with our high-level findings and can teach Team Vittles a great deal more about the local situation outside the Jonathan Alder district.

Lessons learned: partners, planning, persistence, and assistance

If you would like to work on increasing participation in summer food programming at your library, community or state, there are a few recommendations that Team Vittles would like to pass along.

The concept of feeding hungry children is almost always popular, but we have found that it can sometimes be like arguing to erect a prison. People like to have prisons, but "not in my back yard." If you run up against this argument, search out external partners. Community centers, YMCAs, churches are often willing and located in eligible areas. Take the library to them with programming and other forms of outreach.

Start planning early. The State Department of Education and your sponsor, who work together to administer the summer food service programs, are also understaffed, so it may not happen quickly. If you wait for the last second, you may find that children in your neighborhood are hungry for an extra summer. The deadlines for filing your paperwork are generally rolling deadlines, extending from February into summer. Therefore, try to start planning in the fall the year before you want to start. This will give you plenty of time to find a sponsor and make sure your facilities are ready, unless you really want to pay the bills, cook the food, and fill out the paperwork yourself.

Don't try to do it all yourself. In the United States, your state's Department of Education should have an office that works with SFSP. School districts work with the same program for free and reduced-price lunches, and they can often be of assistance in pointing you in the right direction. Several state libraries are involved in SFSP as well. We can also help get you pointed in the right direction. You can find us on the web at http://www.teamvittles.org/.

Don't be afraid to call, email, and knock on doors. The people with whom you are trying to partner are busy, but generally glad to see others focus on issues of concern to them. Many times, they may not respond right away. You may have to make contact several times before you get a response. It is important to note many of these individuals are stretched very thin and are often volunteering after working their day job and tending to their family needs.

In the case of Madison County partnerships, they were successful not because we created something new, but because we found ways to blend in to the existing structure where our job was to fill in gaps.

Steps to develop successful partnerships for lunch **outside** the library.

Visit the USDA's SFSP mapping tools page to determine the eligible areas of greatest need in your service area: https://tvit.us/maptools

Contact your state's responsible agency to find out if there is a sponsor organization at work in your area already. Within the United States, to find your state's agency, please refer to: https://www.fns.usda.gov/sfsp/sfsp-contacts

Having a ready sponsor makes the sales pitch to potential sites much easier: https://tvit.us/sfsptoolkit

Check to see which governmental or non-governmental agencies support these type of initiatives in your community.

Begin mapping the existing resources in your community via contacting the social worker at your local school district, the board of health, or local community center.

Visit these groups with a well-prepared introduction.

Once you are comfortable with your introduction, begin seeking out your community leaders to support the endeavor.

Once you have made introductions, begin determining if your high-level overview of need agrees with the description you're getting from your conversations with your contacts.

Find out if groups that do not show on the USDA maps are at work.

Work with your new contacts to see who is centrally located and likely both willing and able to participate in SFSP.

Approach and select an organization to be a site.

If working with the United States Department of Education, begin connecting site and sponsor early so that the sponsor can get their paperwork in and inspect the site's facilities prior to the beginning of the February application cycle.

Make sure your site is prepared to have a minimum of two adult supervisors for each meal session, along with some alternates in case one is sick or otherwise absent on a given day. Larger sites will certainly benefit from having more.

Children enjoy assisting with such activities and should be encouraged to do so, but regulations require at least two capable adults on site at all times.

Begin connecting the site with organizations that can help provide programming. It is our experience that kids would rather be hungry than bored.

Be prepared to help raise funds if the sponsor requires a deposit to help cover any startup costs or overages.

Be prepared to advertise as much as possible. Have locations, dates, and times ready before the end of school so that information can be sent home with the kids. Tip: Please don't schedule lunch too early. Kids sleep late in the summer.

This process, as described above, can be used in most situations. It was developed using our history working with the Jonathan Alder Local School District, which is largely rural but does have one population center with over 4,000 residents and a good infrastructure currently in place. The process as described will scale up for more urban areas and those communities with a more compact service area, but may not scale as well for service areas that do not have a population center or do not meet the eligibility requirements for SFSP. There are several libraries and communities having great success using bookmobiles, buses, food trucks, and other innovative methods for delivering summer food to rural communities in order to meet these needs.

The team recognizes that hunger takes many shapes and sizes. It can be masked by multiple generations living in the same house, or by families who have found themselves with more house than they can now afford, or by many other acts of ill fate. Team Vittles encourages librarians to be part of the conversation to start anti-hunger services in your communities beyond just SFSP. When the infra-structure does not exist in your community, find those people or be that person who books the library's meeting room and starts the conversation. Look at the needs, the possibilities, and the players in your community and don't hesitate to bring those resources together.

Some Additional Resources:

- Nutritional status of Canadians https://vlc.ucdsb.ca/c.php?g=216719&p= 1434975
- British Nutrition Foundation https://www.nutrition.org.uk/foodinschools/ teachercentre/resources.html
- Nutritional status in Latin America https://www.slaninternacional.org/ images/publicaciones_grls/170912_nutrition.pdf
- CDC Immigrant and refugee health – nutrition https://www.cdc.gov/ immigrantrefugeehealth/profiles/central-american/health-information/ nutrition/index.html

Don't wait for change – feed it.

Team Vittles

References

Children's Hunger Alliance. (2014). 2014 Ohio summer nutrition scorecard. Retrieved from https://childrenshungeralliance.org/wp-content/uploads/2016/12/Ohio-Summer-Nutrition-Scorecard-14.pdf

Madison County Public Health. (2017). 2017 Madison County Community Health Improvement Plan (CHIP). Retrieved from http://madison.oh.networkofcare.org/ content/client/1257/MCPHCHIP2017.pdf

Ohio Department of Education, Office for Child Nutrition. (2017). Data for free and re-duced price meal eligibility: 2017–2018. Retrieved from http://education.ohio.gov/ getattachment/Topics/Other-Resources/Food-and-Nutrition/Resources-and-Tools-for-Food-and-Nutrition/MR81-Data-for-Free-and-Reduced-Price-Meal-Eligibil/ October-2017-Data-For-Free-and-Reduced-Price-Meal.xlsx.aspx?lang=en-US

United States Department of Agriculture, Food and Nutrition Service. (2018). Sum-mer food service program. Retrieved from https://www.fns.usda.gov/sfsp/ summer-food-service-program

20

THE ASK

Partnering to connect at-risk teens with sexual health resources

Elizabeth Lynch and Rebecca McFarland

Can you still get pregnant if you do it in a pool? What are crabs? How do I clean my vagina? These are just a few of the real questions teens submitted anonymously to The Ask, a collaboration between the DuPage County Health Department and the Addison Public Library. The partnership created new points of access for teens and changed the culture around teen sexual health in a resistant community.

Addison is a suburban community with nearly 37,000 residents 20 miles west of Chicago. Addison has the highest teen pregnancy rate in DuPage County with 10.2 births per 1,000 females aged 12–18 (DuPage County Health Department, 2015). Chlamydia rates are nearly double the average for the county as a whole (Illinois Department of Public Health, n.d.). Young people in Addison are also more vulnerable as they are predominantly low-income and from traditionally underserved groups (Centers for Disease Control [CDC], n.d.). In 2017, 67% of children in Addison were classified as "low-income" and 68.4% identified as Hispanic (Illinois State Board of Education, n.d.). The local health clinic reported extremely low usage by young adults, especially males, even though it is centrally located and in walking distance from both the junior high and high school (Millare, n.d.).

These indicators made Addison a priority for the DuPage County Health Department's federally funded teen pregnancy prevention program. In January 2016, the DuPage County Health Department was awarded funding from the Illinois Department of Human Services to reduce rates of sexually transmitted diseases (STDs) and teenage pregnancy. Illinois was one of 84 grantees to receive funding from the United States Department of Health and Human Services, Office of Adolescent Health (OAH) Teen Pregnancy Prevention Program (TPP). TPP is a national, evidence-based program that funds diverse organizations that are working to prevent teen pregnancy.

There are four different types of projects under this funding stream, but the DuPage County Health Department received the five-year, Tier 1B grant, whose goal is to implement evidence-based practices to scale in communities of greatest need. The evidence-based teen pregnancy prevention programs are those proven through rigorous evaluation to reduce teen pregnancy, behavioral risk factors underlying teen pregnancy, or other associated risk behaviors using a holistic approach in safe and supportive environments, in trauma-informed ways, and with linkages and referrals to youth-friendly services.

The primary goal of the grant is to implement an evidence-based, comprehensive sexual health curriculum in the schools during the traditional school day. The co-author who served as the TPP project coordinator began by reaching out to the local school districts, but she met significant resistance. The Addison community is majority Catholic and has a large foreign-born population, making topics like sexual health, especially teen sexual health, culturally sensitive. Most likely, the school believed the integration of sex education into the classroom would result in complaints from parents, board members, and other community stakeholders.

The TPP Project Coordinator turned to other community partners by working with Addison Resources Connect, formerly the Business-Education Partnership Council. The group is headed by the high school and meets monthly to coordinate efforts between government agencies, local-nonprofits, the school districts, and other community stakeholders for young people and their families. After the TPP Project Coordinator presented the grant and its goals, the library representative recommended that she reach out to the library's Teen Services Coordinator, the exemplar author.

The Addison Public Library is located across the street from the local junior high. They serve over 100 students a day using the library as a place to "hangout," do homework, or participate in programs after school. The Teen Services Coordinator was already familiar with the high rate of teen pregnancy and knew anecdotally from working with teens after school that they had few places to turn for accurate information. Because librarians cannot give medical advice or interpret medical information, there were few ways for staff to address this need in a developmentally appropriate way. Those teens that were willing to start a conversation about sexual health topics with a librarian were frustrated that they could not get direct answers. Instead of using the sources librarians directed them to, teens were discouraged from reaching out at all. The Teen Services Coordinator recognized that by partnering with the county health department, the library could connect teens directly to the resources they needed while staying within the ethical and legal bounds of the profession.

The partnership

The partnership began with a pilot of the evidenced-based curriculum supported by the grant. The pilot class met over the summer of 2016 and had an average of 13 participants per session ranging in age from 11 to 17. Students gave feedback on the course, but also served as a focus group for the project partners. They probed the teens for information on what resources they used for health information, who or what they trusted, and what they thought would be effective in fighting teen pregnancy. The answers were often surprising. Students did not want resources online and had a strong preference for face-to-face contact. They also said they were most likely to trust medical professionals, but felt uncomfortable going to a healthcare provider. They wanted information, but they preferred learning through games and discussion. Recognizing a unique opportunity, the project partners used the final sessions of the class to design a resource responding directly to this feedback.

Together, the group built a program called *The Ask*. Inspired partially by the popular US TV program *Loveline*, the program allows teens to ask anonymous questions of a panel of experts that mix humor, advice, and accurate health information. The Ask not only provides information, but also puts a face to local organizations and resources. The project partners reached out to local healthcare providers like the Title X (healthcare) clinic, Teen Parent Connection, and social services for panelists that could form personal connections with teens. These organizations also provide free condoms to participants in discreet bags with informational pamphlets.

Each program begins with a statement from the librarian about anonymity, inclusiveness, and the use of words like "vagina," "anal," and "masturbation." The librarian explains that teens are welcome to leave at any time if they are uncomfortable. The panelists are introduced along with the resources they represent. A list of questions submitted anonymously online in advance is compiled by the teen librarian with minimal editing or censorship. Generally, questions are first asked of the general audience and then turned over to the panel for accuracy and commentary. Participants are given a chance to ask follow-up questions or comment, and discussion sometimes continues among participants, especially if the question is about family or relationships. Periodically, the librarian asked participants to get up and answer a question by walking to an area of the room. This provides an opportunity to move and often sparks further discussion, because attitudes are visible to the entire group. About half way through, the program breaks for pizza, soda, and cookies. Recently, a final game was added to the end of the program, testing participants' knowledge of the information covered at the event. The teen with the most correct answers wins a gift card to a local fast food restaurant. The tone of the entire program was intentionally kept light, encouraging laughter and informal talk between participants and panelists.

Initial outcomes were extremely promising. As of May 2018, 19 sessions of the Ask had been hosted at the library with an average of 20 participants per session. Between January 1st and June 30th 2017, use of the local Title X clinic featured on the panel doubled (Millare, n.d.). The clinic attributed this increase to its outreach at the library.

The project partners hosted a second pilot of the sex education curriculum in the summer of 2017, this time with participants receiving credit for the class at the junior high. The following school year, the district administration agreed to integrate the curriculum into 7th and 8th grade health classes. The partnership has also sparked a broader collaboration between the school districts, the library, healthcare providers, and local social services. These stakeholders formed a committee to develop an online and print resource guide to serve as a comprehensive tool for teens and anyone working with teens. Because of their partnership on the Ask, the library was invited to join the Information and Education Council hosted by the local Title X clinic. The library helped the clinic redesign its website, handouts, and other outreach efforts to be more teen-friendly. Representatives from the clinic set up tables during the library's busiest times with games and incentives to draw teen participants. Most importantly, the pilot classes and the Ask broke the silence on teen sexual health and sparked a culture shift in the community.

Roles

Each partner plays a critical role in the success of The Ask. Funds from the grant awarded to the health department support the panelists, food at the program, and incentives for the final quiz game. Sponsorship by the health department made it possible for teens to receive medical information and resources directly without violating professional and legal standards for libraries. The library intended to use the support of the health department to help justify the controversial program to concerned patrons or board members, though the library has received no complaints. The health department was also essential in finding and securing panelists for the program from local health services, organizations with which the library did not have established relationships.

Comfort and familiarity with teens was essential to moderating the program, especially since the group changes each month. Similar groups of participants would show up sporadically for a few months, but within six months an entirely new group would be attending. The participants range from ages 11 to 19 and had an even greater range of knowledge, experience, and maturity. Teen librarians used their expertise in adolescent development and familiarity with the participants to select questions, students to call on, and topics to discuss. It was essential to create the right atmosphere, balancing humor with trust and authority. As one participant put it,

> The questions were funny in a good way that people was able to laugh at and feel good to be there at The Ask. I loved how they answered questions gently and explaining it. Most people would just be like, uhhhh...look it up online.

Although teens submitted questions anonymously online, this was not sufficient to gauge gaps in knowledge or false beliefs among teen participants. It also provided no way to judge the effectiveness of the events. The project partners began using a quiz game at the end of The Ask in order to assess general knowledge of health information, attitudes on health topics, and impact of the program. For example, 90% of participants at one event answered "Yes" to the question, "Do I need permission to see a doctor." This told the project partners that the overwhelming majority of teens did not know their rights and the resources available to them. From that point on, the panel was instructed to highlight free, confidential medical services available to teens at the local clinic. However, after panelists discussed sexually transmitted diseases, 100% of participants correctly answered the question, "Can you get HIV from a toilet?" The project partners plan to use these quizzes more regularly in the future to track the effectiveness of the program and prioritize topics.

The non-traditional learning environment of The Ask was designed to make up for the absence of a traditional sex education curriculum at the school district. Now that the curriculum has been integrated into health classes, The Ask plays a complimentary role. There is only so much time in any class, health class is only one semester, and sexual health is only one part of the curriculum. The Ask extended the learning in the classroom and connected the information students received to resources in the community. The alternative setting was also an outlet for students that were uncomfortable asking questions in the classroom. An increasing number of questions related to issues of gender and sexual identity, and The Ask has become known as a "safe space" for LGBTQ+ teens.

The project partners were surprised by the disproportionate number of male teens in the program. It's impossible to be sure whether this is due to the model of the program, the content, or some other factor. However, a few teens told librarians that they could not go because they were not "one of those girls," and because parents would not let girls go out at night. This anecdotal evidence suggests that while there were no complaints about the program from community members, conservative values in the community could be limiting its reach.

Recommendations

Because the health needs addressed by The Ask were potentially controversial, it is essential to adapt the model to each community in culturally competent ways. The project partners worked with teens to make the program relevant to adolescents and respectful of cultural norms in the community. For example, teens helped design the flyer for the program, which avoided stigmatizing participants or triggering complaints from parents. Because teens navigate the worlds of both their peers and their parents, they are especially good resources for cultural information. Even for those that are adapting The Ask, working with teens is recommended.

Selecting the right panelists was a central concern for the project partners. Even if organizations provided excellent services and had knowledgeable staff, they needed a teen-friendly representative that could make real connections with the participants. The TPP project coordinator used her knowledge of local organizations to identify representatives that had experience with teens, especially teens in Addison or similar communities. Preference was given to panelists from local organizations, especially in walking distance of the junior high and high school, so that teens met staff they could later contact for help or services. However, in order to provide a complete and engaging panel, representatives were sometimes used from organizations in neighboring suburbs or Chicago. To prepare panelists, the TPP project coordinator discussed the intended tone of the program and common teen behaviors. Those not familiar with teens might mistake the use of a phone or chatting with a friend as disrespect or disengagement, but this type of response was acceptable in the library setting and necessary to make teens comfortable with a taboo topic.

Although the library, the health department, and the school district received no complaints, all three were well-prepared to answer any concerns. Any organization considering similar programs or partnerships should prepare their staff with scripts to respond to potential complaints. Leaders should be similarly prepared to answer to board members, other significant stakeholders, or organized resistance.

While the project partners were able to secure sustained funding for the program, it is possible to replicate the model without funding. Food and prizes were offered because incentives often help draw reluctant teens. However, it is often not the incentive itself, but the role the incentive plays in providing a social explanation. Teens do not have to express interest in sexual health topics, but can convince friends to go for the food or prizes. Credit towards classes in school, volunteer hours, or even teens with excellent social and leadership skills can have the same effect. In fact, the highest attendance at the project partners' events resulted from marketing by popular teen volunteers. Similarly, funds were initially used to pay speaker fees for panelists, but this funding was not necessary to sustain panelist participation. Because government agencies and nonprofit organizations are committed to prevention of teen pregnancy and sexually transmitted diseases, they were willing to send staff to The Ask as part of their regularly scheduled hours. For these partners, The Ask provided a unique opportunity to reach an important demographic with whom they struggled to connect.

Moving forward

The project partners hope that their experience will inspire other organizations in similar communities to address controversial health topics. Resistance from potential partners should not deter organizations from moving forward on projects concerning teen sexual health, drug use, or other taboo health issues. The project partners changed attitudes and brought in skeptical partners by harnessing the resources already available to them and demonstrating success.

The project partners are expanding on the partnership in several ways. The health department is considering spreading the model to more communities, using Q and A events at libraries to address other areas of health disparity. The project partners intend to partner on other health topics, including drug prevention, youth well-care visits, and healthcare enrollment. They are also presenting on the success of the program at professional library and healthcare conferences to encourage more organizations to use the model of The Ask or partner to address community health needs in non-traditional ways (Figure 20.1).

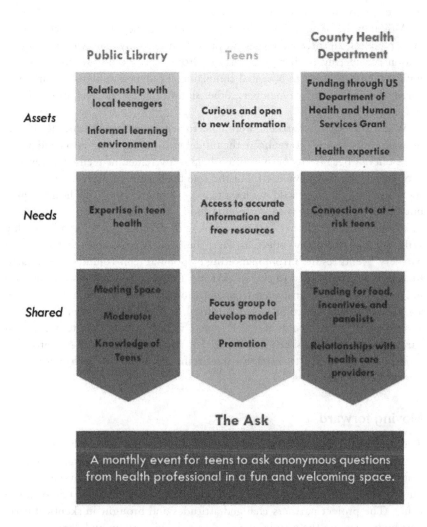

FIGURE 20.1 The Ask.

References

Centers for Disease Control. (n.d.). *Social determinants of health*. Retrieved from https://www.cdc.gov/socialdeterminants/index.htm

DuPage County Health Department. (2015). [Teen pregnancy prevention program fact sheet]. Unpublished raw data.

Illinois Department of Public Health. (n.d.). *IDPH 1990–2016 STD Illinois by County Chlamydia* [Data file]. Retrieved from https://data.illinois.gov/dataset/371idph_19902016_std_illinois_by_county_chlamydia

Illinois State Board of Education. (n.d.). [Interactive Graph] *Illinois report card 2017–2018: Addison school district 4*. Retrieved from https://www.illinoisreportcard.com/District.aspx?source=studentcharacteristics&source2=studentdemographics&Districtid=19022004002

Millare, N. (n.d.). Access community health network title X grant reporting. Unpublished raw data.

21

PHYSICAL ACTIVITY AND LIBRARIES

How library-recreation partnerships contribute to active living

Noah Lenstra

Introduction

This chapter synthesizes North American data on health and wellness programs developed collaboratively between public libraries and parks and recreation departments (henceforth referred to as recreation departments) in order to provide readers with actionable ideas and promising practices. Increasing evidence shows that both public libraries (Whiteman et al., 2018) and recreation departments (Moeller et al., 2017) play critical roles in the health and quality of life in North American communities. Furthermore, recent conference presentations (Gayman & Glaude, 2017), continuing education webinars (Donlan et al., 2018), and magazine articles (Wachter, 2018) illustrate a growing need for support forming and sustaining collaborations between public libraries and recreation departments. For instance, in January 2018 a librarian in the American Library Association's Programming Librarian Interest Group on Facebook asked: "Have any of you experienced successful partnerships between libraries and recreation departments"? The top response (in terms of number of likes) was, "You'll generally find that under either 'fiction' or 'fantasy,' with an occasional episode shelved under 'horror.' Occasionally, you can find it as a happily-ever-after story" (Lenstra, 2018). The perception that recreation departments and libraries don't work well together has also been mined for comedic purposes in the television program *Parks and Recreation*, in which the recreation department continually feuds with the library over local resources.

This investigation into how these two publicly funded institutions collaborate, despite their differences, around the goal of increasing healthy physical activity will serve as a foundation for readers interested in developing similar projects. The context of the reported research project is the World Health Organization's physical activity campaign "Let's Be Active: Everyone, Everywhere, Everyday" (WHO, 2018) which, in response to the health challenges associated with our increasingly sedentary societies calls on new institutions (such as public libraries) to play a more important role in supporting physical activity.

In North America public libraries and recreation departments are components of local government found in virtually every community. This "localness" is crucial because, as the U.S. National Recreation and Park Association states recreation departments "are as diverse as the communities that they serve, and what works well for one agency may not be best for" others (2018, para. 1). The same is generally true of public libraries, of which nearly 90% of funding comes from local tax bases.

How do these two local institutions partner together to support healthy communities? Past work on this topic has focused on programming opportunities and potentialities, but without investigating how those partnerships actually play out. For instance, writing for the Urban Parks Institute, Schull (1998) discusses three ways that libraries and recreation departments can collaborate: (1) sharing their spaces, (2) developing programs together, and (3) collaboratively developing informational services. Schull (1998) identifies that libraries and recreation departments have great affinities:

> [B]oth represent 'the commons.' They are our public space and we hold them together, and they're our collective responsibility. They're part of the underlying urban infrastructure- as important as the bridges and the roads and the housing. They promote civic participation; they foster local identity, and they both offer recreational, educational and social engagement opportunities.
>
> *(para. 6)*

Nevertheless, despite having these affinities, the empirical evidence suggests these partnerships do not naturally form. Writing on a partnership that involved a recreation department partnering with a public library to promote skateboarding as a form of healthy physical activity, Ellithorpe (2018) suggests that one obstacle to forming partnerships is the fact that the two units are so similar, with a great overlap in their functions and roles.

On the library side, the context of this investigation is an ongoing shift in public librarianship towards programming as central to the profession. According to the U.S. Institute of Museum & Library Services (2017), attendance at public library programs increased nearly 35% since 2004, while according to the Public Library Data Service report (Reid, 2017), between 2011 and 2016 "library programs per capita have grown at a rate (6.3 percent) twice the decrease in circulation per capita (-3.0 percent)". In other words, programs at libraries are increasingly central, eclipsing more traditional roles such as circulating collections and reference transactions. In this context, public librarians increasingly form partnerships with other organizations in their communities with whom they may collaboratively develop and deliver programs.

This shift is also aligned with contemporary thinking in the field of public health on the roles of public libraries. In a state-wide survey of how public libraries impact health, scholars from the University of Pennsylvania (Whiteman et al., 2018) found that:

> [L]ibraries also serve as sites of educational health programming. However, among libraries surveyed, patron inquiries generally outstripped programmatic offerings in this domain. This disparity between demand and actual health-related programming offered at public libraries represents a promising, untapped area of need.
>
> *(p. 4)*

To shift into the role of a provider of high-quality health-related programs, public librarians need collaborators to complement their areas of expertise in reading, information, and stories. Recreation departments may be among those collaborators.

Methods

In Spring 2017, public libraries throughout North America were invited to self-select for participation in an online survey on programs they had offered that included physical activity (Lenstra, 2017). Between February 14 and March 23, a self-selecting sample of 1,828 public librarians began the "Let's Move in Libraries Survey", and, among those, 366 responded to the open-ended prompt: "If your library developed these programs and services with partners, please specify who these partners are here". Among those respondents, 129 (35%) stated that partners included recreation departments, making recreation departments the most common partner in North America for this type of health programming.

To analyze experiences of public librarians partnering with recreation departments to develop and deliver these programs, the author analyzed the open-ended responses these librarians gave in response to the survey (see Lenstra, 2017, for a full copy of the survey). Their responses were analyzed using standard grounded theory techniques (Charmaz, 2012), with the goal being to understand how these collaborative programs operated.

Findings

Library and recreation department partnerships do not lead to one particular type of program. Among the more commonly reported programs resulting from these collaborations were: StoryWalks in parks; yoga at the library; summer reading programs in parks; senior, youth, and adult exercise classes at the library; community gardens; storytime activities/events that include exercise; tree, bird, and rock identification walks; and accessing passes from libraries for entrance to recreation centers (i.e. public gymnasiums), parks, as well as checking out recreation equipment (e.g. horseshoes or tennis racquets), hiking equipment (e.g. backpacks), and/or general nature supplies (e.g. birding kits – backpacks with supplies such as binoculars that can be used to enhance one's experiences exploring nature) at the library.

It is also important to note that in some cases collaborations involved partners beyond libraries and recreation departments. One librarian said they did a "walking, hiking program in conjunction with" a public health coalition that involved county parks, state parks, and municipal parks, "all working together to promote more outdoors physical activity". Another identified that their "Libraries Outside" programming series includes partners in the U.S. National Park Service, a regional park, and local recreation departments. A third said that "StoryWalk is a collaboration between multiple entities" in the local community, while a fourth stated the "library operates a Community Garden next to our building. The garden was developed with the recreation department. Anything harvested from the library's garden is placed on a food pantry to serve the community". These examples show that partnerships involving recreation departments and libraries may involve other community partners all working together around shared goals.

In any case, of all the library programs that were developed with recreation departments as a partner, the most common was StoryWalks, reported by 23 libraries. The StoryWalk® concept was developed in the early 2000s by Anne Ferguson with the help of Rachel Senechal of the Kellogg-Hubbard Public Library in Montpelier, Vermont. It involves posting pages of children's storybooks in parks so that families walk together as they read the story. Ferguson came up with the idea while "working in the field of chronic disease prevention .... I wanted to figure out ways to help people be more physically active. I wanted parents as active as children", and she saw the StoryWalk as something that could be "fun, free and something with some substance to it" (quoted in Vogt, 2015, para. 11).

Playing to partners' strengths

More generally, librarians report trying to weave stories into collaborative programs focused on increasing healthy physical activity. For instance, one librarian reported having a monthly storytime at a local recreation center in which, after the story, kids do gymnastics with recreation department's staff. Similarly, another librarian reported that they have a program called "Fit-Lit, which is a partnership with the local recreations centre where-in we have a selection of audiobooks available for rec centre users to sign out and use while doing their workouts on their equipment".

On the other hand, others saw the roles of librarians expanding beyond literacy and stories to also encompass recreation and movement. One librarian stated, "movement is a wonderful thing to promote through libraries", while another said that "our mission statement includes serving the recreational needs of our patrons", so they saw fostering recreational physical activity through things like yoga classes at the library as a natural fit with the library's mission. Furthermore, some librarians defined literacy quite broadly, such as one who stated:

> We believe literacy is an experience of the senses, thus we often try different 'experiences' to add to the understanding of what people are reading or doing. We have used walks to highlight our Big Reads, thus we have [with recreation departments] been in the woods, gone to a neighboring city on the train, walked through neighborhoods, geocaching, etc.

Regardless of how librarians framed their roles in these collaborations, public libraries and recreation departments bring different things to these partnerships (Figure 21.1). Libraries usually offer a free public space open long hours, as well as expertise in stories, information, and literacy. Recreation departments usually offer both outdoor and indoor spaces, which sometimes have entrance fees, as well as expertise in landscape maintenance and recreational physical activity. Partners play to each other's strengths by using the library as a freely accessible space for physical activity and using parks for walking story programs.

A re-imagining of how library spaces can be used stimulates some of these collaborations. One librarian wrote that their library "started offering daily senior exercise programs last year [at the library] and attendance has steadily grown". Here, the library provides the space and recreation departments provide instructors. Similarly, another wrote that "the collaboration and partnership is amazing, especially when you reach out into the community and offer the library space, as a community space, then the sky's the limit" in terms of what types of programs one can do in that space. Another wrote that physical activity programs "promote the idea that the library is a community gathering space ... We are trying to break stereotypes".

To offer these sorts of programs within libraries requires partners that complement the expertise of library staff. One librarian wrote that "whenever we can partner with another institution that can offer expertise, it's a bonus" while another identified that "we are always looking for individuals or groups that are

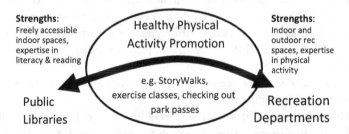

FIGURE 21.1 Empirically derived model of park-library partnerships to increase healthy physical activity.

able to help supply programming ... since we have no programming budget to pay presenters". Others discussed seeking partnerships to cross boundaries. One indicated that "we wanted to see more crossover between departments", which led to recreation departments supporting exercise classes at the library.

In addition to collaborating to develop programs that take place within libraries, librarians also reported working to reduce access barriers to recreation departments facilities. In many communities the library is located either within a park or adjacent to a recreations facility. One librarian recounted that since "we are located in the same building as the park & rec offices", the library worked with them to develop a system wherein library patrons could "check out", or borrow passes to the community recreation center, which normally requires a membership fee, in this way removing a barrier to access. Similarly, a different library found a way to offer a "free pass to the community center" to those who signed up for library cards during "library card sign-up month". Other libraries form partnerships that enable them to offer free passes to state and national parks that otherwise require entrance fees.

Libraries also take their expertise out to recreation departments facilities. One wrote that by having off-site storytimes at recreation centers they combine "literacy with physical health at the children's level" while another wrote that "partnering with the recreation center is great to introduce health aficionados to the ways that reading can be combined with their physical activities". Another library developed a program called "Barks and Books: A book discussion that takes place at a dog park where owners bring their dogs to exercise during the discussion". Others mentioned walking book clubs that meet in area parks. StoryWalks, of course, also fit within this trend.

Challenges and lessons learned

Partnerships do not always go as planned, and in some cases collaborations were abandoned. Obstacles reported by librarians include: not enough time, assessment difficulties, and legal and logistical hurdles. Partnerships do not form themselves. In the busy environment of the public library, finding time to initiate and sustain partnerships was, for many, a challenge. One librarian wrote the partnership "take[s] initiative and energy from other programs". Another stated it was challenging to "schedule staff for outreach events". A third stated that "coordination with parks departments took a long time", while a fourth wrote that "working with recreation department" was the biggest challenge associated with this type of programming.

Librarians also reported difficulty figuring out how to assess these collaborative endeavors, especially those that take place outside the library. One wrote that "our StoryWalks are self-guided so it is hard to know how much they are used". Another wrote that "although it's not very quantifiable, we do receive good feedback from the community and our partners". A library with a summer reading program focused on getting residents to visit and walk in local parks found their "biggest issue is getting the report mechanisms back – we know people participate, but we find it hard to get the things back that indicate the type and amount of participation". A library with a similar program wrote: "patrons did it on their own time, I have no way of tracking except by how many points sheets were turned in at the end of the program". These quotes illustrate a need to develop easy-to-implement assessment techniques for these programs.

Finally, legal and logistical challenges plagued some partnerships. Legal issues centered around concerns about the library being held liable in case of injury. One wrote that securing "approval to take underage participants off library grounds" was a challenge. Another stated that securing "permission slips to take kids to the park" and "developing an appropriate waiver of liability for adult hiking programs" posed difficulties.

These programs also created some general logistical headaches for librarians. A library that offered Zumba and Jazzercise through a partnership with recreation departments said that "due to the noise of the music and the space needed we could only accommodate [these programs] in a community room". At other locations, staffing changes at recreation departments led to difficulties. Librarians discussed fitness instructors retiring or leaving the recreation departments, which left libraries with disruptions in their schedules. Another librarian talked about how "staffing changes" in the National Park Service led to constraints in a program focused on circulating park passes at the library, as the library lost their contact who had handled all the logistical matters within the park service.

Transportation and weather issues also created obstacles. One library ultimately abandoned a collaborative community garden program because the "gardens are not within walking distance to the library". Another wrote that the "whole set up proved to have a lot of research needed", more than was initially anticipated. One librarian said that participation in a weekly librarian-led walk in the park "has been HORRIBLE" because of the weather. Another said they had to cancel programs due to "inclement weather", while another stated that "cooperative weather conditions" are essential to outdoor programs. For instance, one librarian stated that "lows down to -45C restrict when and how we can offer programming" while, on the end of the spectrum, a different librarian stated that "heat in the middle of the summer" deterred participation. The weather also affects the sustainability of StoryWalks, with librarians reporting challenges with the "fading of materials", the "wind blows them away", and not knowing "how do we maintain the signs?" One librarian wrote that due to the "weather effects on the StoryWalk pages, we did not repeat this" program.

In other cases, however, lessons learned from these challenges led to deepened partnerships. For instance, librarians reported learning to let recreation departments handle the maintenance of the supplies associated with StoryWalk programs, since that is their area of expertise. One wrote that library staff "pick the stories and update the signholders" while the recreation departments staff take care of the physical maintenance of the displays. Another wrote that recreation department's staff "help with winterizing the signs and replace them if vandalized". In these examples, libraries and recreation departments have learned to play to their respective strengths, forming effective partnerships that knit together physical activity promotion with literacy and reading.

Benefits and outcomes

Despite the challenges associated with assessing these collaborations, librarians did report positive outcomes such as strengthened communities and an improved perception of the role of the library in terms of the quality of life in the community. A librarian who worked with recreation departments to bring yoga to the library wrote that "people comment positively on the wide variety of quality services offered" at the library. Another wrote that a similar collaboration "planted a seed – we often get requests now for more yoga programs". Another wrote that the library's "teen advisory board often asks for these types of programs", and the library tries to fulfill these needs through partnerships with recreation departments. In addition to strengthened communities, these programs also contribute to health. One librarian wrote that in their community "our public school cut recess time, and in the face of all the research that shows kids need to move their bodies (we all do)" they found that collaborative programs with recreation departments were positively contributing to community members making "healthier physical choices".

More generally, collaborations contribute to building bridges across different sectors of the local community, contributing to a cohesive quality of life. A librarian wrote that a story time/physical activity program at the recreation center has

> allowed [both] the library and recreation departments to gain new users. I have seen more parks participants at library programs and they [library patrons] also enrolled in sports programs at recreation departments. This has become our favorite program at the library.

More generally, and despite challenges, librarians tend to frame collaborations with recreation departments in positive terms. One librarian "left a waterproof booklet and sharpie for people to comment" at the end of their StoryWalk in the park and "the response was overwhelming".

Discussion

Forming and then sustaining programming partnerships between public libraries and recreation departments takes time. For many, the results warrant this investment. Despite challenges, most respondents reported satisfaction. In addition, at a time when librarians are increasingly called to practice "networked leadership" to become "community catalysts" (IMLS, 2016), librarians need to find ways to recognize and valorize the work that goes into forming and sustaining these

TABLE 21.1 Practical lessons from investigation

Lessons	Public Library	Recreation Department
Know what each partner brings to the partnership	1. Facilities open to the general public without entry costs 2. Expertise on stories, information, and literacy	1. Parks and recreation centers (not always free) 2. Expertise on physical activity and nature
Build on strengths of partners	Example of StoryWalks: Librarians maintain stories	Example of StoryWalks: Recreation department maintains display apparatus
	Example of exercise classes: Librarians maintain free, open space	Example of exercise classes: Recreation department provides instructors
Have contingency and assessment plans in place	Partnership should be institution to institution, and not individual to individual: If an individual leaves, the partnership continues. Assessment mechanisms developed/ shared among partners.	

types of partnerships. It is true that this energy takes time away from other work, but it is also true that both libraries and recreation departments can have larger impacts on the quality of life in their communities by working together.

An example of these lessons coming together in the real-world emerged as this chapter was going to press. In Delaware, the Dover Public Library "is working hand-in-hand with parks and rec to offer a multitude of recreational and educational programs" during the summer months (Finney, 2019, para. 8). The "Tuesdays in the Park" program emerged from a shared realization that both institutions needed to do more to extend access to their respective services, beyond libraries and recreation centers. Each program includes literacy components led by the library, physical activities led by the recreation department, and free meals provided by the Delaware Department of Education. Each partner has clear responsibilities that play to their strengths, and assessment is incorporated into the project plan. During the first year, they discovered that families wanted to check out books, so in the second year the Kent County Public Library started bringing their bookmobile to the programs. Table 21.1 includes general lessons broadly applicable from this study, all of which are seen in this example. Key points include: (1) know what each partner brings to a partnership, (2) build on those respective strengths, and (3) have contingency and assessment plans in place.

Conclusion

Ending what public health scholars call the global pandemic of physical inactivity requires a multi-sectoral response. It is for this reason that the World Health Organization's (2018) physical activity campaign is called "Let's be active:

Everyone, everywhere, everyday". The idea that only one sector of society has responsibility for increasing physical activity is increasingly outdated. Public libraries can and do have a role to play. This chapter illustrated how libraries can answer the call by forming and sustaining partnerships with recreation departments. More research and hands-on work are needed to help us understand how to form, develop, sustain, and assess these and other health-oriented community partnerships.

References

Charmaz, K. (2012). *Constructing grounded theory.* Los Angeles, CA: Sage.

Donlan, E., Henson, D., Reopelle, R., & MacDonald, M. C. (2018). Public libraries and community partners for wellness literacy. *Kernel of Knowledge NNLM Webinar Series.* Retrieved from https://nnlm.gov/class/public-libraries-and-community-partners-wellness-literacy/8081

Ellithorpe, C. (2018). Learn to skateboard: Partnering for health and exercise. *Programming Librarian.* Retrieved from http://www.programminglibrarian.org/blog/learn-skateboard-partnering-health-and-exercise

Finney, M. (2019, May 28). Hot fun in the summertime: Dover Parks & Rec set for busy season. *Delaware State News.* Retrieved from https://delawarestatenews.net/news/hot-fun-in-the-summertime-dover-parks-rec-set-for-busy-season/

Gayman, D., & Glaude, N. (2017). *Partnering with your park.* Paper presented at the meeting of the Association for Rural and Small Libraries, St. George, Utah. Retrieved from http://bit.ly/NOLS-PARK

Institute of Museum & Library Services (IMLS). (2016). *Catalyzing communities through stronger leadership.* Retrieved from https://www.imls.gov/blog/2016/10/catalyzing-communities-through-stronger-leadership

Institute of Museum & Library Services (IMLS). (2017). *Public libraries in the United States survey: Fiscal year 2014.* Retrieved from https://www.imls.gov/sites/default/files/publications/documents/plsfy2014.pdf

Lenstra, N. (2017). Movement-based programs in US and Canadian public libraries: Evidence of impacts from an exploratory survey. *Evidence Based Library and Information Practice, 12*(4), 214–232. doi:10.18438/B8166D

Lenstra, N. (2018). Parks & Rec: A health programming partner. *Programming Librarian.* Retrieved from http://www.programminglibrarian.org/blog/parks-rec-health-programming-partner

Moeller, A. M., Andersen, J., Van Den Elzen, J., Gemignani, R., & McMullen, S. (2017). Evolving role of parks and health care to collaboratively enhance public health: A practitioners' perspective. *Recreation, Parks, and Tourism in Public Health, 1*, 75–79. doi:10.2979/rptph.1.1.06

Reid, I. (2017, September/October). The 2017 public library data service report: Characteristics and trends. *Public Libraries.* Retrieved from http://publiclibrariesonline.org/2017/12/the-2017-public-library-data-service-report-characteristics-and-trends/

Schull, D. D. (1998). Parks and libraries in partnership. *Great parks/great cities 1997–1998.* New York, NY: Urban Parks Institute. Retrieved from https://www.pps.org/article/schull

U.S. National Recreation and Park Association. (2018). *NRPA park metrics.* https://www.nrpa.org/publications-research/ParkMetrics/

Vogt, T. (2015, July 14). In StoryWalk, kids run to the page. *The Columbian*. Retrieved from http://www.columbian.com/news/2015/jul/14/storywalk-kids-run-to-next-page-hazel-dell/

Wachter, R. (2018, January). Out of the branches, into the woods: Libraries and state parks collaborate on hiking backpacks for patrons. *American Libraries*. Retrieved from https://americanlibrariesmagazine.org/2018/01/02/hiking-backpacks-branches-woods/

Whiteman E. D., Dupuis R., Morgan A. U., D'Alonzo B., Epstein C., Klusaritz H., & Cannuscio, C. C. (2018). Public libraries as partners for health. *Preventing Chronic Disease, 15*, 1–9. doi:10.5888/pcd15.170392

World Health Organization. (2018). *More active people for a healthier world: The global action plan on physical activity 2018–2030*. Retrieved from http://www.who.int/ncds/prevention/physical-activity/gappa

SECTION D
Capacity building

22

INTRODUCTION

Building community capacity through partnerships and collaborations

Henry R. Cunningham

Oftentimes communities are tasked with providing services that are beyond their capacity because of lack of resources or perhaps the lack of expertise is absent. Such situations require communities to collaborate with other entities to provide the services to their residents. Consequently, partnership is an important aspect of capacity building. It allows the partners to collaborate where each brings its own set of resources or expertise (Mohamad et al., 2013) to address a common cause. Capacity building is defined differently depending on the entity but there are still underlying similarities in the definitions. The National Council of Non-profits define capacity building as "an investment in the effectiveness and future sustainability of a nonprofit". Another definition by Enemark and Ahene (2002) states that capacity building is development of human resources to develop and maintain certain aspects of society. What is common about these two definitions is the investment in human capital to ensure sustainability over time. This is important for community success as it takes human and financial resources as well as time to have any true impact in addressing community needs. Capacity building is the focus of this section of the book. Various authors present projects that focus on building individual and community capacity to address needs that exist in communities.

Kelley and Sulzychi from the Springfield City Library in "Hoop City Blooms Mason Square Community Garden and Public Health Initiative" detail how the library partnered with several entities to convert a vacant lot, used as a dumping ground, into a community garden of vegetables, complete with park benches for residents to enjoy the outdoors. The purpose of their project was to build health literacy and work toward alleviating food insecurity in the community. Besides having a place to plant and harvest fresh vegetables, the project also provides gardening workshops, programs on nutrition, free seeds, and soil testing and a green space in a parklike setting.

What is unique about this project is that these librarians realized they could not accomplish all this on their own. They sought out interested partners, who had the resources and expertise to provide meaningful assistance. They sought out the Parks and Recreation Department to offer advice on constructing a community garden and the Springfield Food Policy Council to provide guidance on food literacy, among others. Three different categories of partners played a role in the success of this project: those who were initial contributors, funding partners, and the program and activity partners. This project clearly provides a blueprint for those interested in undertaking such an initiative in their community.

Building capacity involves educating others on topics of significance to ensure sustainability over an extended period. Armed with such information can alter one's life outcomes. Informed individuals make better decisions based on the knowledge they have, which consequently affects life outcomes. In "Patient Empowerment: A Partnership between Academia, Community-based Organizations, and Public Libraries", the authors set out to empower individuals in the community with new information, which subsequently affected their decision-making and choices made. This partnership that included academia, community-based organizations, and public libraries embarked on a project to educate individuals with whom they worked, on how to access online health information and how to prepare for an appointment with their healthcare providers as well as how to interact with that person during the appointment. Having this knowledge enabled these individuals to be more informed about health matters and to be better advocate for their health.

In order to build capacity extensively, this project entails empowering caregivers and public librarians with information as well. To ensure sustainability public librarians, who were providing information on accessing health information to those who frequented the library, were provided with the necessary information and certification to continue educating individuals who visit the library. The goal was for library visitors to have continued education.

The concept of capacity building is of even more importance in rural communities, particularly in developing countries where resources and facilities may be lacking. In such instances, project sustainability is key to ensure long-term impact. Rogers, Torres, Uribe, and Young through their respective organizations partnered with others to address deep rooted beliefs and traditions that had adverse effects on rural communities in Bolivia and Ecuador. Child Family Health International, based in San Francisco, California in the United States, partnered with a hospital in rural Bolivia to create the Young Women Empowerment Project, aimed at providing young women with health information and training to combat years of cultural beliefs and tradition that was negatively affecting the health and wellbeing of young women. Projects of this nature bring significant challenges because they require a cultural shift within the community, which may take a long time to occur.

While the project in Ecuador in which Child Family Health International embarked was not as culturally imbedded in the community, the community health programs implemented still required significant education and imparting of knowledge to change individuals' lifestyles on health-related matters. Both programs required navigating significant cross-cultural differences, which could only come through sensitivity to the community's culture. This section speaks of the importance of providing cross-cultural training for individuals who chose to work in communities such as those in Bolivia and Ecuador, where cultural practices are distinctly different from those of individuals working in these communities. It is important to be respectful of and be sensitive to others culture and be aware of cultural conflicts that may arise.

Tarver, Dobbins, Olmstadt, Duggar, and Esparza provided an overview of several projects on which they embarked that enhanced the capacity of individuals to be more effective in their community. They illustrated how different teams collaborated with each other to design a symposium for librarians and first-responders on how to deal with threats of suspicious persons and active shooters; to create online resources for parents, teachers, and healthcare providers; and a health literacy project among others. The authors detailed how the various partners collaborated to ensure the success of the projects as well as the contribution of each partner. They noted issues involved in collaborating with others to build capacity as well as steps taken by the group to ensure success. Of major importance is the need to have clearly delineated roles and responsibilities for each partner. Funding for the projects was key as they identified how they were funded through grants.

These chapters give us an overview of several projects to build individual and community capacity. They provided detailed steps that led to project development and implementation through collaboration for those who may want to engage in similar initiatives. The challenges encountered and lessons learned are important for those pursuing similar projects. The pitfalls encountered in these projects are great lessons for others on what they should avoid.

References

Enemark, S., & Ahene, R. (2002). Capacity building in land management—Implementing land policy reforms in Malawi. *Survey Review, 37*(287), 20–30. doi:10.1179/003962603791482875

Mohamad, N. H., Kesavan, P. K., Razzaq, A. R. A., Hamzah, A., & Khalifah, Z. (2013). Capacity building: Enabling learning in rural community through partnership. *Procedia – Social and Behavioral Sciences, 93*, 1845–1849. doi:10.1016/j.sbspro.2013.10.128

National Council of Non Profits. (n.d.). What is capacity building? Retrieved from https://www.councilofnonprofits.org/tools-resources/what-capacity-building

23

HOOP CITY BLOOMS

Mason Square Community Garden and Public Health Initiative

Caitlin Kelley and Ellen Sulzycki

Introduction

Farming and local produce are quintessential parts of Massachusetts' Pioneer Valley culture, though you might not know it while walking through the neighborhoods surrounding Springfield's Mason Square. The neighborhood lies at the intersection of four of Springfield's smaller neighborhoods, Bay, McKnight, Old Hill, and Upper Hill. The combined neighborhoods are incredibly diverse, the majority of its residents being people of color. In 2012, the Pioneer Valley Planning Commission noted that 38.25% of people in Mason Square are living below the federal poverty line, only 3.25% of residents have easy access to affordably priced, healthy food, such as vegetables, fruits, and whole grains, and just 10.5% of residents have obtained a bachelor's degree (Data Atlas). The factors that influence the socioeconomic position of individuals and groups, such as education, income, and race, also influence their health (Centers for Disease Control and Prevention, 2013).

While it may be the place where James Naismith invented basketball by tossing a ball into a peach basket, the neighborhood is named after 19th century black entrepreneur and abolitionist, Primus Mason, who left most of his fortune to benefit poor, old men in his community. Unfortunately, generations of urban decay have left this area blighted and the soil contaminated with lead. The Square contains numerous fast food chains and bodegas, but residents have almost no access to healthy food options.

The environmental and socioeconomic factors residents face, as well as lack of access to proper nutrition, disproportionately affect residents' health. In order to address these health issues, the librarians at the Mason Square Branch of the Springfield City Library have endeavored to foster an environment of health-conscious, community-oriented, and sustainable living through building

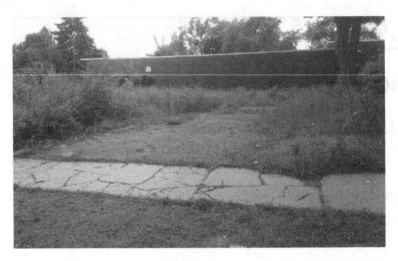

FIGURE 23.1 View of the vacant lot beside Mason Square Branch Library.

a foundation of health literacy and working toward alleviating food insecurity. The library, alongside nearly a dozen community partners, provides the local community with gardening workshops; nutrition programming for youth and adults; free organic seeds and soil testing; community garden plots and green park space; and access to trustworthy health resources (Figure 23.1).

This project grew organically and gradually. It began in April of 2014, with a community member reaching out to their local library. A Mason Square neighborhood resident and president of Springfield's Stone Soul Music Festival visited the Mason Square Branch Library. The resident suggested to the reference librarian that the library clean up the lot alongside the branch and host an event for families in the summertime in the space. This particular lot was flanked by the library's two parking areas. It consisted of a crumbling driveway, shoulder-tall weeds, and the kind of garbage typically found on un-stewarded city land. Eager to do something constructive with the space, the librarian agreed to this proposal and met with the resident and other representatives from Stone Soul to discuss the details of the community event, which they scheduled for the end of the summer.

Following the meeting of representatives from Stone Soul, the librarian discovered the perfect opportunity: Outside the Box, a grant program funded by Redbox and managed by Online Computer Library Center (OCLC) in partnership with Projects for Public Spaces. The mission of the Outside the Box program was to turn unused outdoor spaces into community event spaces. The Springfield neighborhood of Mason Square was one of 22 communities across the country that was awarded this grant, which included training on place-making principles; consultation; reusable materials, including tents, cafe sets, and umbrellas; as well as funding for trees. In light of the award, the Springfield Parks and Recreation Department agreed to remove the old driveway on the lot and cut back all the

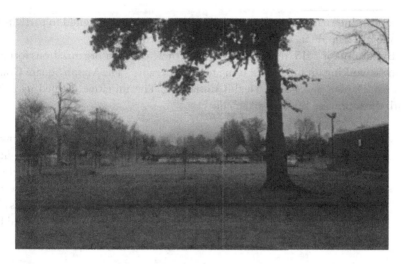

FIGURE 23.2 View of the cleared lot beside Mason Square Branch Library.

brush. The Mason Square Branch Library's first annual Community Festival, attended by almost 300 residents, was held on the library's front lawn. For the summer of 2014, it was moved to the lot (Figure 23.2).

After the cleanup and festival, the lot was no longer used as a dumping ground, but it certainly was not a vibrant community space. The Parks and Recreation Department told the library any further improvements to the space would have to be funded by grants or outside organizations.

Concurrently, a local group of community gardeners had settled into a new garden space a few streets over from the Mason Square Branch Library. They had received a grant to install a water pump in their new space. Sun-loving vegetables, like tomatoes, would not bear fruit on this land, however, because the lot did not get enough sunlight. The gardeners inquired with Mason Square Branch's librarian about the newly cleared lot next to the library in the hopes of placing a new garden there.

Excited about the possibility of transforming the vacant lot to support community gardening efforts, but uncertain of how to proceed, the reference librarian sought guidance and input from local community gardening and health organizations. The Community Garden Coordinator at the Springfield Food Policy Council offered support, as did the Outreach Librarian at Baystate Health, a non-profit health system headquartered in Springfield. One of the Parks and Recreation Department's project managers was enlisted by the library director's office to explore the feasibility of setting up a community garden on city-owned land and to determine how a garden could be incorporated into a larger park space. The librarian set up a few idea sessions with the representatives from the Springfield Food Policy Council, Baystate Health, the city, community gardeners, and members of the library's management team to discuss a community garden and park plan. In follow-up meetings, the Director of Public Health at

American International College (AIC), in Springfield, was invited to participate in order to help further identify community health needs.

By autumn of 2015, representatives of all these different organizations formed a single working group, contributing to what became "The Mason Square Community Garden and Public Health Initiative." The initiative defined its goals with the following mission statement:

> The Mason Square Branch Library and its partners seek to foster an environment of health-conscious, community oriented, and sustainable living by simultaneously constructing a set of community garden plots; developing on-site seed and tool lending libraries; orchestrating an on-going series of gardening, health, and nutrition-focused workshops and activities for both children and adults; and outfitting a safe park space to be enjoyed by all local residents.

The goals set forth by that group formed the basis of Mason Square Branch Library's grant writing and programming initiatives. The first series of grant proposals focused on transforming the lot into a safe, green park and community garden space as well as the establishment of a seed lending library. In addition to the Out of the Box grant, the library received funding from a Lowe's Community Partner grant and a donation from High Mowing Organic Seeds, respectively. Nine raised beds were built on the lot and the space was landscaped, hardscaped, and furnished with benches to create a beautiful, functional park space, where residents and gardeners could gather and enjoy the outdoors. A library of seeds was displayed in a prominent location within the library where patrons could pick out free herb, vegetable, and flower seeds to take home and plant.

To support the health aspect of the Mason Square Community Garden and Public Health Initiative, the Mason Square Branch Library's reference librarian and children's librarian applied for a community engagement grant through the National Library of Medicine (NLM). The proposal submitted to NLM aimed to advance health literacy and aid in alleviating food insecurity in the Mason Square neighborhood. The Mason Square Branch Library received this funding in autumn of 2016 and the success of the first round of programs led to the grant being extended through the spring of 2018. The grant itself, titled "Health In The Square," was made up of four distinct parts: training for librarians, technology implementation, nutrition workshops, and gardening workshops. This grant also funded the purchase of first-time gardener kits and soil test kits that were distributed to community gardeners. The first-time gardener kits included gardening gloves, gardening containers, and a spade. The soil tests, which are processed by the Stockbridge School of Agriculture at the University of Massachusetts in Amherst, educate residents about the potentially detrimental contents of the soil in their gardens. The risk of lead exposure is heightened in urban environments, where

TABLE 23.1 Project partners

Initial contributors: *These partners originally came together to brainstorm the logistics of starting a community garden, seed library, and health programming for the Mason Square Community*

Mason Square Branch of the Springfield City Library	American International College's School of Public Health
Springfield Food Policy Council	Mason Square Community Garden Group
Baystate Health	Springfield Parks Department

Funding partners: *The health initiatives undertaken by Mason Square Branch Library could not have been possible without generous support from sponsors*

National Library of Medicine	Outside the Box
Massachusetts Master Gardener Association	Lowe's Charitable and Educational Foundation
Hudson Valley Seed Company (in-kind donations)	High Mowing Organic Seeds (in-kind donations)

Program and activity partners: *Partners from local community groups and organizations support library programming and health initiatives*

American International College	Springfield City Library Volunteers
Mason Square Health Task Force	Martin Luther King Jr Family Services
DeBerry Elementary School	Springfield Food Policy Council
Muhammad Mosque #13	Community Support Institute
Local chefs	

the historic use of lead in gasoline, paint, and various industrial processes continues to contaminate households, soil, and air. One potential pathway for lead exposure and/or poisoning can be consumption of produce grown in lead-contaminated soil (Knapp et al., 2013).

Many positive results come from these initiatives. Patrons take home kale, onions, strawberries, and other fresh produce harvested from the community gardens. On "Tasty Tuesdays," children and their families create delicious and nutritious no-cook recipes using fresh ingredients. Local gardeners have a space to grow vegetables in soil free of toxins, giving residents free vegetables. Library staff members have been trained to use health resources more effectively. Through multiple projects, the Mason Square Branch library is doing its part to support the health needs of the community by engaging residents in educational, health-related, no-cost workshops, activities, and programs (Table 23.1).

Partnerships

The library's partnerships developed organically. The residents expressed the neighborhood needs and librarians reached out to collaborate with local gardening and health specialists. By collaborating with groups and individuals in the Mason Square neighborhood, the library ensured that efforts were in tune with resident health and cultural needs. It was and continues to be vitally important that the initiative draw as much as possible from the expertise and experience available in the community rather than exclusively relying on outsiders. This allows patrons and programming participants to learn from persons with whom they share lived experience.

The Outside the Box grant provided initial clean-up of the lot, including removal of debris left over from the lot's previous occupants and general litter, commonly found in vacant, urban areas. Following the conclusion of the grant, a working group of residents and non-profit representatives collaboratively generated a list of initiative goals and brainstormed about potential stakeholders, partners, and funding sources. As funding was awarded (from the Lowe's Charitable and Educational Foundation, the Massachusetts master Gardener Association, Hudson Valley Seed Company, and High Mowing Organic Seeds), the focus of the initiative shifted from planning to implementation. The initial contributors to the project stopped meeting as a regular group and instead group members helped the library carry out programming associated with their particular specialty.

The Springfield Food Policy Council's Community Gardening Coordinator, who herself is a Mason Square resident, was instrumental in helping the group identify community needs and resources; as well as directing the development and implementation of community gardening workshops. The Mason Square Community Garden Group participants maintain the garden's nine garden beds and promote community gardening through outreach and by leading educational workshops.

Representatives from Baystate Health and American International College (AIC) connected both the library and community gardeners with a rich network of health professionals. Public health students from AIC, student interns from the Mason Square Health Taskforce, and Springfield City Library volunteers have co-facilitated programs, promoted health resources, and gained valuable field experience. In addition to playing a formative role in shaping the direction of the initiative, the Outreach Librarian at Baystate Health facilitated health literacy training for Springfield librarians and, in her current role as Outreach Coordinator for the National Network of Libraries of Medicine (NNLM), has assisted with administering the Health In The Square grant. Training on reliable, trustworthy online health resources was provided to local area health professionals and librarians, expanding the reach of library's offerings. These partnerships have maximized the project's impact.

Funding from the NNLM for the Health In The Square Grant provided more opportunities for partnership. The library facilitated youth nutritional workshops, "Tasty Tuesdays," with local children from DeBerry Elementary School and Martin Luther King Jr. Family Services. By collaborating with these groups, library staff ensured attendance to their programs and expanded library outreach to new groups. Finally, local chefs became stakeholders for the library and the health programs by co-facilitating nutrition workshops for adults and children including "Tasty Tuesdays."

Outcomes

Tangible results from this health initiative have not been measured because of limited ability to reach out and follow up with program participants. Unfortunately, it is impossible to report if residents who were involved are exhibiting better health. The lasting impression of the Mason Square Community Garden and Public Health Initiative on the health and wellbeing of the residents may be measured in years to come in a Community Health Report.

With the resources available, the measured outputs have been overwhelmingly positive. In the last 3 years, over 100 families have borrowed nearly 1,200 packets of seeds from the seed library to grow their own vegetables. More than 60 first-time gardener's kits have been distributed to local residents for gardening at home. Nine residents, four representatives from the local mosque, library staff, and a dozen non-profit mentor/mentee pairs from an organization working with at-risk youth have successfully grown and consumed a variety of vegetables in the community garden. Community garden members and librarians have twice been invited to represent Springfield at the Northeast Organic Farming Association's Summer Conference.

Library staff members have also reported a decrease in alcohol use and drug activity on the lot since the project started. In previous years, drug paraphernalia and empty alcohol bottles were found frequently on library grounds. Since the outdoor lighting was installed, and the park was built on the lot, there has been a lesser degree of evidence related to wrongful activity on library property.

Finally, attendance of programming associated with the initiative has also been strong. To date: 166 children attended 11 youth nutrition workshops, 266 adults and children attended 16 gardening workshops and events, 17 adults attended three nutrition programs, and 13 librarians and community health professionals were trained in NLM health resources.

This project resulted in valued partnerships across the Mason Square community, the City of Springfield, and the State of Massachusetts. Not only did the library benefit, but so did its project partners. Some gained a greater knowledge of the community's needs and of ways to fill those needs. Project participants developed gardening and coalition-building skills. Project partners gained both social and professional networks.

Lessons learned

1. **Demonstrated commitment is infectious**. A number of gardening program participants decided to get involved after seeing library staff or community garden members working in the garden picking tomatoes and watering the plants. For example, the local mosque and members of a mentoring program both inquired about what was happening in the garden and subsequently joined in on gardening the next season.
2. **Working on a big team can elongate projects**. While all municipalities are different, the process of getting approval to develop public land often requires input and coordination from multiple officials and/or departments. Working

with a variety of non-profit organizations to make sure that the needs of the community are met in addition to defining project goals takes time.

3. **Momentum is easily lost.** It takes consistent, active involvement to keep stakeholders motivated and involved. While trying to attain the full potential of a project, adherence to protocol can elongate the timeline and setbacks may cause a team to lose energy. Poor project execution can result in minimized outcomes and may depress a team as well. These discouragements can be learning experiences. It is important to have a plan, refresh your goals frequently and break down big projects into realistic steps to keep energy up.

4. **As projects evolve, so do the roles of partners.** Some partners may take a more active role in the project, some may take a step back. As projects evolve, goals might be amended and partners' involvement may change. For example, the head of AIC's Public Health Department was instrumental in helping the library identify the health needs of the community and the appropriate programming to respond to those needs; however, his role changed during the programming implementation period. When nutrition programming for children was implemented, AIC provided student interns from the Health Department that were available to assist with the programs, but the department head himself was no longer actively involved.

5. **Working in a city neighborhood facing very high rates of poverty and crime comes with its own set of challenges.** It was expected that

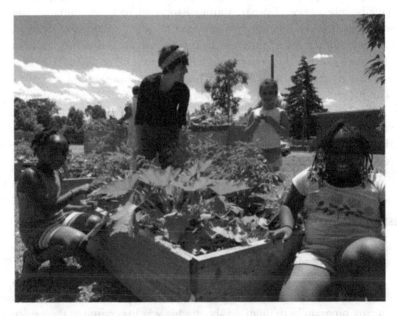

FIGURE 23.3   Librarian Caitlin Kelley and three young library patrons tend to one of the community garden beds.

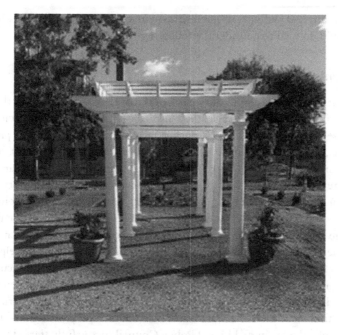

FIGURE 23.4 View of the completed park space, with community garden boxes visible in the background.

people would take vegetables from the garden. It was not expected that people would use the garden hose to wash their clothing, would steal whole containers of plants, or use drugs while hiding in the bushes. Subsequently, a surveillance camera and motion lights have been installed in the area to deter any serious crime. A proposed tool lending service was discontinued due to potential liability issues (Figures 23.3 and 23.4).

Recommendations for starting a community garden

While the librarians at the Mason Square Branch Library and their partners have worked on the Mason Square Community Garden and Public Health Initiative for years, applying for grants, fostering community connections, and setting up programming, this type of initiative can be scaled up or down, depending on community needs and available resources.

Setting up a community garden requires little money, but a lot of sweat equity, which means that the project can easily be replicated, as long as there are enough people to keep it going. Before a library (or non-profit, community group or intrepid individual) begins its own community gardening adventure, they would do well to consider the following:

Community need and interest

The great thing about community gardens is that they not only fulfill the body's need for fresh, healthy produce, they also can provide individuals with a way to engage with their community, engage in physical exercise, model pro-social behaviors, and generally make people feel happy that they are a part of something positive. Just because there is a need, however, does not necessarily mean that there is an interest. A lot of people like the idea of a community garden, but when it comes to such tasks as constructing raised beds, hauling compost, or watering on a 100-degree (Fahrenheit) day in August, the idea may lose its luster.

Gauge interest in your community: reach out to the leaders in the neighborhood, the people who have the pulse of the community, who are helpers, and to whom residents look up. If you cannot take the time to set up a focus group, create an informal survey asking who in the community could both benefit from and be willing to commit to a community gardening project long-term. Alternatively, find out if there is a captive audience with whom you might collaborate. For example, the Springfield Food Policy Council successfully started two community gardens by working with resident groups at the local housing authority.

Location and water access

The garden should be located in a sunny spot with easy access to water. Many vegetables require six to eight hours of direct sunlight each day to bear fruit. If land is not readily apparent, consider organizations (schools, churches, or community centers) that have extra space that might be shared and could themselves benefit from a community garden. Alternatively, you can find out if there are vacant, city-owned lots that might be used with permission from the city.

Awareness of soil toxins

If you are planning on gardening in the ground, have the soil tested first to make sure that the soil is not contaminated with lead or other dangerous heavy metals or pollutants. Many universities have labs that process soil tests for a nominal fee. If access to a soil test is impossible, use containers or lined raised beds to prevent the possibility of soil contamination.

Time, money, and handy people

The costs of purchasing pre-made raised beds, bagged compost, and vegetable seedlings from your local nursery can add up quickly. If funding is limited, then creative thinking will be essential in order to keep expenses low. Luckily, there exists no shortage of books or online articles on how to transform scrap materials (tires, pallets, soda bottles) into plant containers. That said, pulling apart a pallet and reconfiguring it into a garden box takes time and skill. It is important to balance priorities and be realistic about what kind of projects a group can undertake.

Conclusion

Over the course of four years, librarians working at the Mason Square Branch Library in Springfield, Massachusetts collaborated with community-based organizations, city workers, educational institutions, and local residents to try and address the neighborhood's lack of healthy, accessible produce and the prevalence of poverty-related health disparities. By developing a community garden and park area, the library and its collaborators have provided a space where residents can relax, enjoy being outdoors, and grow their own food at no cost. Series of gardening programs provide resident gardeners with the knowledge necessary to grow safely, healthy and bountiful crops. Nutrition programming gets children excited about eating healthy foods that they can make by themselves and instructs adults on amending existing diets to combat diseases such as heart disease and diabetes. Free seeds, from the branch's seed library, encourage residents to start their own garden, whether it is in their yard or in a flowerpot on their windowsill. Collectively, these programs promote health in the community and abolish the assumption that the library is merely a repository of books; it is a place where people come together to learn, create, and grow (Table 23.2).

TABLE 23.2 Timeline of mason square community garden and public health initiative

Mason Square Community Garden and Public Health Initiative	
Due Date	*A Timeline*
April 2014	Patron expresses need for more community events/ clean-up of branch's blighted lot
August 2014	First Community Festival, funded by Outside the Box, attended by 300+
March 2015	Community gardeners reach out
March 2015–April 2016	Partnering, brainstorming, planning, outreach, brainstorming, grant writing
April 2016	Seed library opens
May 2016	Community garden beds planted
August 2016	Lowe's Community Foundation Grant funded
October 2016	Health in the Square, NNLM Grant funded
November 2016	NNLM resource training for librarians
2016–2018	Tasty Tuesdays program serves 116 kids
April 2017	Massachusetts Master Gardener's Grant funded for community outreach
May 2018	Springfield Garden Club partners to make pollinator garden and workshop

References

Center for Disease Control and Prevention. (2013). CDC health disparities and inequalities report, *62*(3). Retrieved from https://www.cdc.gov/mmwr/pdf/other/su6203.pdf

Knapp, L., Sangster, J., & Bartelt-Hunt, S. L. (2013). The influence of lead hyperaccumulators on the uptake of lead by vegetables. *International Journal for Service Learning in Engineering, Humanitarian Engineering and Social Entrepreneurship, 8*(2), 1–7.

Partners for a Healthier Community, Inc. (2014). Springfield health equity report: Looking at health through race and ethnicity. Retrieved from https://www.publichealthwm.org/application/files/7315/1568/8099/1610815-PHC-Health-Equity-Report_web.pdf

Pioneer Valley Planning Commission. (2012). Data Atlas [map]. Retrieved from http://pvpc.maps.arcgis.com/apps/MapAndAppGallery/index.html?appid=6ef5baa0e3e9435a865d5a4a81e38ca7

24

MAKING AGENCY FUNDING WORK FOR YOUR COMMUNITY

Talicia Tarver, Montie' Dobbins, William Olmstadt,
David Duggar, and Julia M. Esparza

Academic health sciences libraries are in unique positions to help promote health literacy in their communities. As employees of research institutions, health sciences librarians can thus leverage their partnerships with clinicians, researchers, and local nonprofit organizations to create health literacy programming relevant to the members of the community (Whitney et al., 2017). Academic health sciences libraries also have access to unique funding opportunities through the National Network of Libraries of Medicine (NNLM, *Funding Opportunities*, 2018a). These funding opportunities are further specialized by region, depending on where the academic library is located. With its location in Shreveport, Louisiana, the Louisiana State University Health Shreveport (LSUHS) Health Sciences Library (HSL) is part of the South Central Region (SCR) (NNLM, *Regional Medical Libraries*, 2018c). The SCR has access to funds dedicated to consumer health outreach, health literacy, and disaster preparedness, to name a few (NNLM, *Funding Opportunities*, 2018a). It is with this funding, LSUHS HSL implemented several projects over a six-year period that were designed to achieve the same goal: to give local members of the community access to quality healthcare information.

For many of the projects (see Table 24.1) at LSUHS, the HSL devised a variety of strategies to provide health education, tools, and resources for our partner organizations. Classes, train-the-trainer sessions, and symposia have put our project partners and their audiences in touch with useful resources. Equipment such as televisions, computers, and printers have made it easier for people to share and access health information. Projects have resulted in creative deliverables our partners can use, including graphic novels for children, patient education materials related to Human papillomavirus (HPV), mental health checklists and manuals, and web portals to help users access online resources. Regardless of the

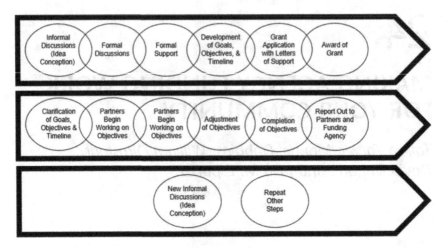

FIGURE 24.1 Funding development cycle.

projects' deliverables, the foundational goals and objectives for all of them was to provide the surrounding community with access to quality healthcare information that was properly vetted by experts (see Figure 24.1).

Generally, the awards discussed in this chapter were completed during a one-year funding cycle, as they are awarded by the NNLMSCR. However, projects truly begin when the funding opportunities are announced, approximately one to two months before application deadlines. Librarians meet to discuss ideas and potential partners and then approach partners to see if they are interested in collaboration. Only after all project partners agree does the application process begin. From beginning to end, many projects may last 14–16 months, and successful collaborations sometimes result in future projects.

Projects begin in a variety of ways. Sometimes a librarian already has a partnership with a colleague or an organization because of past collaborations. It is not unusual for the nature of an award, such as the Disaster Preparedness Award, to inspire an idea based on a previous project. Sometimes a librarian is simply passionate about a need within the community and uses these potential collaborations to address that need. Therefore, LSUHS HSL librarians generally propose program ideas to community partners with whom they have previously worked on other health literacy or community engagement projects. Once the community partners are on board with the proposed program ideas, the librarians apply for funding through NNLMSCR.

LSUHS HSL has successfully applied for and received award funding for many years, although not every project submitted has been funded. The projects featured in this chapter highlight a variety of partners that have ranged from a private practice outpatient medical office to state-wide agencies. These projects focus on a specific six-year period, 2012–2018, rather than the entire history of

TABLE 24.1 Projects, partners, and funding agencies

Project	Dates	Partners	Type of Partner	Funding Agency	Amount Funded
Promoting the Environmental Health Student Portal (Student Portal)	2012–2013	Caddo Parish School Libraries Supervisor (CPS Libraries) Caddo Parish School Science Supervisors (CPS Science)	Public school	National Network of Libraries of Medicine South Central Region (NNLMSCR)	5,000
YMCA of Northwest Louisiana Project (YMCA)	2012–2013	YMCA of Northwest Louisiana (YMCANWLA)	Nonprofit community organization	NNLMSCR	20,015
Disaster Preparedness Award: Are You Prepared? (Prepared)	2013–2014	Northwestern State University College of Nursing & School of Allied Health Shreveport Campus (NSU) State of Louisiana Department of Health Office of Public Health Region 7 (LADH Region 7) Bossier Parish Libraries (BPL) Shreve Memorial Library (SML) Centenary College of Louisiana (CCL)	Academic institutions State agency Public libraries	NNLMSCR	10,000
Do I Need to Worry? Mental and Developmental Checklists for Parents and When You Need It (Do I Need to Worry)	2013–2014	LSUHS Department of Psychiatry (LSUHS Psychiatry) Caddo Parish School Psychologist (CPS Psychologist) LSUHS Children's Center (LSUHS Children's)	Academic medical departments Public schools Academic outpatient clinic	NNLMSCR	25,000

(Continued)

Project	Dates	Partners	Type of Partner	Funding Agency	Amount Funded
Health Literacy Comic Book (Captain Fit)	2014–2015	LSUHS Department of Pediatrics (LSUHS Pediatrics) LSU Shreveport Department of Arts and Media (LSUS)	Academic medical department Academic institution	NNLMSCR	5,000
Intruder Alert: A Symposium on Suspicious Persons, Active Shooters, and Threats to a Library (Intruder)	2015–2016	NSU LADH Region 7 CCL	Academic institutions State agency	NNLMSCR	8,000
Shreveport Medical Society Alliance Health Project Grant (SMSA)	2016	LSUHS Pediatrics	Academic medical department	Shreveport Medical Society Alliance (SMSA)	1,565
Teaching Science through Gamification: Promoting Education on Health Topics within the Caddo Parish School System in Northwest Louisiana (Gamification)	2016–2017	CPS Libraries CPS Science	Public school	NNLMSCR	10,000

LSUHS HSL award funding. The purpose of these partnerships has always been to create teams of librarians and those who would benefit from and would promote the goals of the project. Generally, the LSUHS HSL librarians chiefly functioned as project managers and/or principal investigators after securing funding for the project, while the community partners provided subject expertise, venues for events, and access to members of the community. Partners often taught alongside librarians, but in instances where librarians were the chief creators of materials, partners served as consultants to ensure that the information was medically and ethically correct before submitting their approval for the final product.

The following examples illustrate how teams on the projects have worked in various ways. These examples are from projects named in Table 24.1. For example, in Intruder Alert, LSUHS HSL collaborated with Northwestern State University (NSU) and Centenary College of Louisiana (CCL) libraries and the Louisiana Department of Health Office of Public Health (LADH) Region 7 to design a symposium to educate academic, public, and school librarians and first-responders on the protocol for dealing with threats of suspicious persons and active shooters. The partners worked closely with LSUHS HSL to identify the speakers for the symposium, to develop materials to be handed out to participants, and to provide the logistics for the symposium. In the project Meeting the Community Information Needs Regarding Human Papillomavirus (HPV) Vaccinations, not only did the team work together to develop goals and materials, the academic medical departments and state agency provided personnel to speak during the conference to help educate the community. For other projects, the roles of LSUHS HSL and partnering agencies were a little more delineated, as with the Young Men's Christian Association (YMCA) of Northwest Louisiana (NWLA) project for which the team met at the beginning to determine what materials would be promoted in order to meet the goals. It was then up to the LSUHS HSL librarians to develop materials, to set up tables, to promote the objectives, and to interact with the individuals entering the facilities. In the projects involving public schools, the schools were active developers of the material to better serve their community of science teachers and librarians. In some instances, authority from the clinical sites was necessary to ensure that materials were displayed or distributed, as with the Shreveport Medical Society Alliance (SMSA) – Health Project Grant. The success of all projects was due to the symbiotic relationship between the librarians and community partners, each lending their specific skill sets and (in the case of the partners) their authority to ensuring the program reached the desired target audience.

Each project resulted in strengthening partnerships that are still perpetuating opportunities and materials to further help the community access reliable consumer health information. Tangible outcomes that resulted from these partnerships can be categorized as either Internet-based information, event participation, or equipment purchased to help an organization better educate community members.

Internet-based information includes the Teacher Education web page, created as part of the Teaching Science thru Gamification project with the corresponding resource manual, *Teaching Science thru Gamification: Resource Manual of Educational Games linked by the National Institutes of Health* (NIH) and bookmarks of online educational games by grade school and science discipline. LSUHS HSL also created a web portal for educational mental and developmental resources for parents, teachers, and healthcare professionals, and helped to increase the visibility of the National Library of Medicine's (NLM) *Environmental Health Student Portal*. LSUHS HSL's involvement in an HPV educational symposium led to the library's creation of files for participants to easily print and make additional copies. LSUHS HSL partnered with LSUHS Pediatrics Department to create *Captain Fit*, a youth-appropriate online comic book on adopting and maintaining healthy nutrition and lifestyle.

In addition to creating online resources, LSUHS HSL also applied for funding to cover the expense charged by the Medical Library Association (MLA) for granting certification in MLA's Consumer Health Information Specialization (CHIS). GeauxConsumerLA promoted and provided access to free online courses for Louisiana librarians, library staff, and other information professionals to fulfill the MLA CHIS requirements. Other events coordinated through NNLMSCR funding mentioned previously in this chapter were the Intruder Alert symposium funded through a Disaster Preparedness Award and the HPV Symposium funded through a Consumer Health Outreach Award.

LSUHS HSL also worked with the local YMCA NWLA to provide brochures for online health resources and other items (wristbands, towels, pedometers) to participants in Kids Triathlon, YMCA Half Marathon and 5k, and Urban Adventure Race. The YMCA NWLA also allowed the HSL to hold classes on online health information for a variety of ages, including Broadmoor After School (middle school) students and Gray Panthers (senior adult) members. Finally, NNLMSCR funding was used to purchase computers and printers for two YMCA NWLA locations so that members could look up links to NLM resources that were listed in the brochures. Logs were also left by the computer stations to document how often members accessed information through these computers. In partnership with LSUHS Pediatrics Department, LSUHS HSL used Shreveport Medical Society Alliance (SMSA) funding to purchase two monitors placed in pediatric clinical settings. These monitors allowed patient education materials to play in waiting rooms.

Challenges and lessons learned

These projects would not have succeeded without the support and cooperation of the community partners as well as the creativity of the HSL librarians in meeting challenges inherent in coordinating such projects, no matter the size of the project or the involvement of community partners. Even so, coordinating these projects presented challenges. Budget, equipment, timing, staff, promoting awareness and participation were the universal challenges librarians faced while completing these projects. When outlining the budget for a project, it is important to determine which partner's organization might be the better fit for receiving and managing the funds. Even in a partnership within the same institution, as in LSUHS, the LSUHS Pediatrics had an account system in place to receive and spend funds from the SMSA, unlike LSUHS HSL. In planning for the first Disaster Preparedness Award project, Are You Prepared, LSUHS HSL had an easier accounting process than the two public library systems. As academic institutions, NSU and LSUHS had similar accounting processes, which worked well when NSU wanted to take the lead role in managing the second Disaster Preparedness Award project, Intruder Alert.

Equipment is also a big issue in planning a grant proposal. In the Disaster Preparedness Award, items allowed in the first submission (which was not funded) were no longer allowed when the proposal was re-submitted in the next funding cycle. Flash drives had to change into bookmarks for content delivery. Camcorders and books could be easier to find in vendor catalogs and purchased with institutional credit cards, rather than shopping for televisions in retail stores.

Technical equipment is always a challenge, especially when trying to make something accessible online to anyone anywhere. Bandwidth and speed to access resources in rural areas and firewalls that institutions may have in place can make viewing a recorded program or live participation difficult. The length of a recording can also be a limiting factor. In GeauxConsumerLA, each individual online consumer health course provided by LSUHS HSL using WebEx was capped at one hour in response to technical limitations.

Project staff may be difficult to find, hire and pay as learned when creating the Teacher Education webpage and the *Captain Fit* web comic. When deciding to outsource an aspect of a project, it may be better to line up the outside contractor before submitting the grant application. Having a contractor identified in advance can help ensure that both the funding agency and the partner handling the received funds are able to resolve issues in hiring and paying contractors, as well as accessing equipment onsite or offsite beforehand. It is important when developing projects that at least one partner has access to information technology personnel to handle technology-related problems. All the grants discussed in this chapter had at least one if not two information technology faculty or support staff that were available to handle technology issues.

Community organizations like YMCA NWLA, Bossier Parish Library (BPL), and Shreve Memorial Library (SML) are able and willing to schedule programs at their facilities. However, promoting these activities to draw an audience can be a struggle. Most people go to the YMCA to exercise, not to hear a health talk, and public library branches have different audiences. Tying a program to the meeting time of home-school or daycare visits worked much better than just placing a date on the branch library's calendar. The weather can also derail a program (people stay home in flash flood and tornado warnings).

Project developers must also be aware of each partner's holiday and work schedule during a funding cycle and of fixed dates and deadlines in the project's timeline. In the Promoting the Environmental Health Student Portal (Student Portal) project, the original timeline concluded in the award cycle's seventh month with presentations on how the Student Portal was used in the classroom at the Joint Louisiana Science Teacher Association (LSTA)-Louisiana Association of Teachers of Mathematics (LATM) Conference. Therefore, all classroom programming needed to be completed and conference proposals needed to be submitted by the fifth month. It was therefore crucial to have fixed dates and deadlines to ensure the success of the Student Portal project.

One must also juggle the availability of speakers, facilities, and optimum time(s) to reach the target audience when scheduling a symposium. While all three came together perfectly for the Intruder Alert symposium, the best date for the symposium on Meeting Community Needs Regarding HPV Vaccinations ended up not being the best date to reach the largest audience. A symposium was dropped from the Do I Need to Worry? Mental and Developmental Checklists for Parents and When You Need It (Do I Need to Worry) project, and the focus was instead placed on creating the manual and promoting the resources. This ability to adapt and remain flexible can be the key to a successful project.

Project staff are not always able to accomplish a goal due to outside influences. Materials created on HPV could not be written at a third-grade reading level due to the term "human papillomavirus." There was no way to describe aspects of HPV in lower level words. Other outside influences can include a change in policy between the time of grant application and time of approved grant implementation. This can lead to changes in the concentration of the project.

Partners need to clearly delineate and understand roles and responsibilities. A key supporter of GeauxConsumerLA did not advocate the program to public librarians across the state. The project's staff, therefore, had to put a lot of time into Social Media to raise awareness and encourage participation. YMCA NWLA administration was on board, but staff did not always seem to be aware of Library staff activities. It may thus be necessary to create written agreements or memorandums of understanding between partners, whether in-house or external.

One should not assume you know what the community partners want and need. For example, the better audience for the Student Portal was at the Environmental Education Symposium. The Caddo Parish School (CPS) Science Supervisors focused on low-tech online games accessible to all rather than ones available from apps. Lesson plans to go with the online educational games would have made the Teaching Science Through Gamification project more useful to both the school teachers and the students.

Recommendations

For those wishing to replicate or conduct similar projects, the most valuable recommendations are to communicate, to be flexible, and to continue to show up at community or partner's events. It is important to become recognizable and approachable, as this can encourage potential partners to approach the librarian as opposed to the librarian approaching the partner. While one should never make assumptions, one should be willing to lead and provide support when someone else wants to submit and manage the project. Overall, one should be open to new ideas and new partners or participants before and during the project.

When looking at funding agencies and their awards, one should not limit oneself to those who traditionally fund library projects. A partnering organization may open a new area of funding in which the library can play a role. Knowing what can be funded, both via the funding agency's award requirements and via the library partner's institutional policies, can help set the appropriate parameters for the budget. Contracts may need to be negotiated in advance. Therefore, it is important to find out the costs of all equipment to be purchased or rented and the costs for creating products and materials. Once everything is outlined in the budget, a principal investigator can then reduce and reevaluate the budget until it reaches the set proposal figure. Alternative sources for funding should also be assessed, when necessary, to offset the proposal's stated figure. For example, if the proposal calls for planning a symposium, the costs for recording the speakers for later viewing should also be considered. Partners or other community organizations and businesses can sometimes help with such additional funding.

Another crucial step is to create a timeline for the project with key due dates and deadlines. The timeline should include extra time for setbacks and unexpected events. If possible, the principal investigator should also create secondary plans. Even if alternative plans are not possible, librarians should still remain flexible and allow for change, which is always a constant.

Other examples of flexibility include being open to different methods of programming. Lectures and hands-on exercises may work for some programs, but utilizing a game, interacting with animals, puppets and "characters" can be just as effective. One can also ensure training for the trainers is built into the timeline if working with a software or online product with which librarians or partners are unfamiliar.

Everything should be documented for the required reports to the funding agency. Project managers need not be afraid to ask for changes during the implementation of the project, as funds may need to be moved from one fund line to another due to changes in costs, or due to an unexpected opportunity. Methods of project evaluation vary. A symposium or lecture may have a questionnaire at the end. A new product may have a usage counter with comments or a log recording in what ways the product was used in a school setting by course or classroom. If the project timeline in the funding cycle only has time for creation of the product, the timeline can be adjusted to allow for evaluations along with the steps in product creation. These could be meeting notes or reviews of trials or tests in determining what to include in the product or how the product was working.

As stated, the chief funding source for LSUHS HSL is the NNLMSCR, which is a regional office for the NLM. Unless otherwise specified by the regional offices of the NNLM, funding is available to "institutions whose role includes providing access to authoritative health information" (NNLM, *Health Literacy Award*, 2018b). Many community agencies provide authoritative health information without libraries. They could partner with each other, or with a nearby health sciences library or public library, in efforts to obtain this funding. This broadens the applicability and availability of this funding. Smith (2000) notes that the NLM remains largely unknown to the United States public. Its funding programs represent a potential source of support for community agencies that often goes untapped.

When considering writing grant proposals, it is important to know the community you will serve. We used a group of statistical tools to back up the need for any project. For instance, per United States Census Bureau *QuickFacts* about Caddo Parish, Louisiana (where Shreveport is located), 49.4% of the population identified as Black or African American alone, and 26.4% of the population is estimated to be in poverty (2017). In addition, Caddo Parish, according to *Statistical Atlas* of the United States Census Bureau, has a significant percentage of the population who report Mexican and Vietnamese ancestry (2015). All the funding represented in this chapter was obtained with the idea that authoritative health information could mitigate health disparities. While it is difficult to prove that cause-and-effect relationship, the funding was secured to address health needs that disproportionately affect lower income, international, or otherwise disadvantaged populations. Given the economic and ethnic diversity in Caddo Parish, it is very likely funded outreach programs from this library reached at least some low-income and non-U.S. born citizens.

LSUHS HSL has been very fortunate in its access to award funding and the partnerships acquired over time to create projects that were both effective and appreciated. However, none of the projects would have begun without the librarians' and partners' creativity and initiative to determine memorable ways to meet the community's health information needs. Any library, large or small, can foster their staff's creativity by encouraging librarians to research their target community and the agencies that provide outreach to the community. Identifying these audiences and their needs can lead to ideas for which librarians can play a specific role – especially if the librarians are well-versed in sources of award funding. Once librarians have fleshed out an idea and pinpointed a funding source, they may find any number of agencies willing to partner with them for projects that will leave far-reaching impact on local and surrounding communities.

References

NNLM. (2018a). Funding opportunities. Retrieved October 30, 2018 from https://nnlm.gov/funding

NNLM. (2018b). Health literacy award. Retrieved October 30, 2018 from https://nnlm.gov/scr/funding/health-literacy-award

NNLM. (2018c). Regional medical libraries. Retrieved October 30, 2018 from https://nnlm.gov/regions

Smith, K. A. (2000). From Billings to Lindberg: A continuing story of discovery. Proceedings of the Computers in Libraries Conference, *15*, 252–253.

United States Census Bureau. (2015). Statistical Atlas-Ancestry in Caddo Parish, Louisiana [Table]. Retrieved from https://statisticalatlas.com/county/Louisiana/Caddo-Parish/Ancestry

United States Census Bureau. (2017). QuickFacts-Caddo Parish, Louisiana- Race and Hispanic Origin and Income & Poverty. [Table]. Retrieved from https://www.census.gov/quickfacts/fact/table/caddoparishlouisiana/PST045217

Whitney, W., Keselman, A., & Humphreys, B. (2017). Libraries and librarians: Key partners for progress in health literacy research and practice. *Health Literacy: New Directions in Research, Theory and Practice, 37*, 415–432. doi:10.3233/978-1-61499-790-0-415

25

PATIENT EMPOWERMENT

A partnership between academia, community-based organizations, and public libraries

Kara Burke, Elizabeth Irish, Enid Geyer, Ingrid Allard, Linda Miller, Maria Buhl, and Lauren Manning

Background

Health literacy and the ability to find reliable health information online is important to achieving good health (Devine et al., 2016). A 2003 study found that more than 77 million US adults have basic or below basic health literacy skills (Kutner et al., 2006). Populations most likely to experience low health literacy include older adults, racial and ethnic minorities, people with less than a high school degree or a GED certificate, people with low income levels, non-native speakers of English, and people with compromised health status (Institute of Medicine, 2004). Low levels of education, literacy, and health literacy have been linked with poor health, poor healthcare utilization, increased barriers to care, and early death (Pleasant, 2014). Low health literacy also impacts patient-physician communication. Effective patient-physician communication results in better health outcomes (American College of Obstetricians and Gynecologists, 2014).

Americans increasingly turn to the internet for their health information. In a 2012 survey conducted by the Pew Research Center's Internet & American Life Project, 72% of internet users said that they had looked online for health information within the past year. Seventy-seven percent of online health seekers said that they began their last session at a search engine (such as Google), and 13% began their session at a site that specializes in health information (such as WebMD) (Fox & Duggan, 2013).

The Capital District is a diverse area that includes urban, suburban, and rural communities, with over 800,000 residents spread over four counties. The population varies widely in terms of socioeconomic status, education level, and race/ethnicity, with a large refugee and elderly population (United States Census Bureau, 2017). As previously noted several of these groups are at high risk for low health literacy. The area is fortunate to be served by a complex network of social and educational services, including public libraries, local government organizations, institutions of higher education, CBOs, and medical providers.

Recognizing the need to improve health literacy, patient–physician communication, and the use of online health resources, leadership within SLHS and DivCOME were engaged in ongoing discussions regarding ways to use their respective interests and expertise to address these issues in the local community. The 2016 Outreach to Consumers Award from the National Network of Libraries of Medicine Middle Atlantic Region (NNLM MAR) was the impetus for SLHS and DivCOME to formalize plans and recruit additional partners. DivCOME approached community partners based on the target audiences they hoped to reach as well as on organizational missions that overlapped with the project goals. Each partner has a shared vision to improve health within the community by improving health literacy, fostering patient–physician communication, and providing community health education. This project provided the opportunity to combine the talents of academic institutions, CBOs, and libraries.

Project partners and roles

Key partners

Academic partners

Albany Medical College: AMC, founded in 1839, is one of the nation's oldest private medical colleges. The College is part of Albany Medical Center, northeastern New York's only academic health science center with a mission of providing excellence in education, biomedical research, and patient care.

SLHS, a NNLM MAR resource library, facilitates access to biomedical information resources that support the mission of the organization. Library faculty teach within the curriculum and offer independent consultation and instruction.

DivCOME aims to improve the health of patients, particularly those from ethnically diverse and disadvantaged backgrounds, while educating medical students, residents, and other healthcare providers, utilizing the principles of non-biological determinants of health as the underpinnings of all activities. DivCOME oversees the AMC medical student Service Learning requirement, which is executed through strong relationships with many community partners.

Community-based organization partners

Community Caregivers: Founded in the Albany County Village of Altamont in 1994, Community Caregivers' mission is to enable individuals of all ages to maintain their independence, dignity, and quality of life within their homes and communities. Their services are provided without charge by an extensive network of dedicated volunteers. Client services include transportation, shopping, friendly visits, caregiver respite, light chores, assistance with paperwork, and telephone assurance calls. They find that non-medical services can make or break someone's ability to live independently.

Community Caregivers also sponsors community education sessions aimed at older adults and family caregivers often in partnership with local libraries. As family caregivers shoulder much of the responsibility for informal care, keeping them well is critical to their loved ones remaining at home and not in higher levels of care. Education programs geared to wellness in older adults have included: fall prevention, hearing loss, and the Health Engagement and Literacy Project.

Center for Law and Justice: The CFLJ, founded in 1985, serves the low-income and disadvantaged communities of New York through education and advocacy. The CFLJ is guided by the mission of working to achieve a fair and equitable justice system that values all human life as equal and precious. They primarily serve individuals who are re-entering the community after being incarcerated, but also work to support those who are facing challenges due to poverty, homelessness, substance abuse, and other issues.

Community outreach is crucial to the work conducted by the CFLJ. Through partnerships with organizations such as AMC and the Albany College of Pharmacy they work to identify health issues prevalent in their community and implement effective interventions. This includes community workshops, Law Enforcement Assisted Diversion, and one-on-one assistance addressing health issues.

Public library partners

The Capital District has three public library systems that span the region. Libraries were selected as partners because they serve diverse populations in close proximity to AMC, CFLJ, and Community Caregivers. Albany Public Library and Troy Public Library are urban, Guilderland and Voorheesville are suburban, and Berne serves a rural community in the Helderbergs on the western edge of Albany County. Another library, Rensselaerville, was included as they partner closely with Berne on other projects.

The partner libraries have missions to provide quality library materials and services to their communities for lifelong learning, cultural enrichment, and enjoyment. The public library partners provide varying degrees of consumer health programming. Past program topics include exercise, disease prevention, health education, and patient advocacy. Guilderland Public Library offered a consumer health reference service providing more in-depth health research.

Each partner was critical to the overall success of this project. Project staff were selected from within each organization based on professional interests, skill, and past collaborations. For example, the SLHS instructor holds a Level II Consumer Health Information Specialization (CHIS) from the Medical Library Association (MLA). This specialization requires continuing education in consumer health resources, technology, and services. The Outreach & Education Coordinator at Community Caregivers worked with DivCOME on Service Learning and has strong skills in planning and publicizing outreach events with a network of local partners including public libraries such as Guilderland. The project contact at Guilderland Public Library had a prior interest in providing consumer health information to patrons. The librarian received and maintained the CHIS designation.

The academic partners at AMC, SLHS, and DivCOME were responsible for overall project design, administering grant funds, creating and teaching community workshops, creating and teaching professional development workshops, and evaluation activities. Community partners were responsible for reviewing and providing feedback on workshop content, arranging workshop sites, and promoting the workshops to the targeted audiences. Public libraries were responsible for recruiting a group of librarians to attend continuing education (CE) workshops and ultimately receive CHIS designation. The public libraries each hosted and promoted a community workshop during Phase 2 of the project *(see Chart 1)*. NNLM MAR provided essential financial and administrative support. MLA worked with AMC to obtain CE credits for the professional development workshop and CHIS designation for the public librarians, which served as an incentive for their participation.

Project goals and purpose

The project was completed in two phases. Funding was received for both:

- Phase 1: Community Engagement (Summer, 2016–Spring, 2017)
- Phase 2: Librarian Professional Development and Community Engagement (Spring, 2017–Spring, 2018)

Phase 1: community engagement

The initial phase of the project was working with CBOs. Community-based workshops were developed and delivered by SLHS and DivCOME with input from the CFLJ and Community Caregivers, the latter two organizations advertised the workshops.

The workshops aimed to inform participants how to research health information online, communicate with their healthcare providers, and prepare for a medical appointment. Concepts focused on the importance of asking your doctor questions and using reliable health information sources to help build those questions. A total of 8 workshops were delivered to 54 participants. Settings included a low income senior housing community room, a community learning center, as well as two public libraries. These were intentionally located in urban, suburban, and rural communities. Groups most at risk for low health literacy were targeted. Workshop materials were developed with attendees' varied levels of literacy in mind.

Phase 2: librarian professional development and community engagement

The success of Phase 1 led to the idea of building a sustainable model by tapping into what the public libraries do best – reaching into their communities on an ongoing basis. During Phase 1 of this project, Community Caregivers connected with the two public libraries as sites for community workshops. The partners observed that the workshops held in these two libraries had high attendance rates and levels of participant engagement, which signaled the need for a continuing partnership. Subsequent discussions with the host librarians also identified the need for professional development opportunities in consumer health information. As with choosing the community workshop sites, the partner libraries chosen for Phase 2 represent urban, suburban, and rural communities.

AMC designed an MLA-approved CE workshop, *Patient Empowerment: Using Information Resources to Improve Health Communication,* which built on the content of the community workshop as further incentive for the public librarians. Two additional MLA CE workshops were offered so that 20 participating librarians at 6 libraries were eligible to receive CHIS designation using a fee waiver purchased through grant funding. A total of 25 librarians attended at least one of the workshops. The community workshops developed in Phase 1 continued to be taught at participating public libraries.

Funding

NNLM MAR funding was secured for this project by AMC. In Phase 1 funding, Community Caregivers and CFLJ received subcontracts to help support their time and effort. As some of the community workshop sites did not have computer labs, a traveling projector and screen were purchased to provide more mobility. Laptops and iPads were purchased for use for hands-on practice during the community workshops. In Phase 2, public libraries received iPads to allow them to work directly with patrons away from the busy reference service point, due to the confidential nature of health information. Funds supported the purchase of 20 Consumer Health Information Specialization designation fee waivers from the MLA as well as CE course approval and associated fees.

Outcomes

Significant and sustained partnerships were fostered during the project period and continue into the present. DivCOME had existing relationships with Community Caregivers and the CFLJ prior to the start of Phase 1, but partnering on this project allowed these organizations to work together more closely and expand the scope of services provided to the community. SLHS librarians, who had not previously engaged with these organizations, formed professional collaborations, shared expertise and resources while learning about the services and skills of the CBOs. AMC continues to collaborate with Community Caregivers and CFLJ. These sites host medical student internships and service-learning programs. They are likely to host or facilitate community health workshops in the future.

During Phase 1, eight interactive workshops were offered to 54 participants. We collected 38 pre-questionnaires (70% response rate) and 36 post-questionnaires (67% response rate). Responses to the workshops were very positive, with the percentage of community participants indicating that they are "Very Confident" or "Confident" in their ability to find good, high-quality health information on the internet going from 25% in the pre-questionnaire to 91% in the post-questionnaire. Ninety-seven

Without good health, those we serve, their families and their communities suffer from additional hospitalizations, poorer outcomes, and more complex health needs. Finally, without community supports - including the education and patient empowerment tools offered by projects like this one, individuals we serve in the community are likely to move to assisted living or skilled nursing care facilities sooner than they would with proper supports. The longer we keep older adults successfully in the community where they want to be - the better for everyone involved.

FIGURE 25.1 Community caregivers project impact statement.

percent indicated that they intended to tell a family member/friend about the websites from this workshop. One-hundred percent indicated that after this workshop they will be more comfortable explaining concerns with their physician, and 97% felt that the workshop improved their ability to ask questions at their next appointment. Community Caregivers Outreach and Education Coordinator commented that this project reinforces how simple, direct, and well-thought through messages and strategies can have a positive impact on the health of others (see Figure 25.1).

During Phase 2, AMC strengthened partnerships with local public libraries, creating a sustainable model to continue consumer health information education. This project also provided a venue in which public libraries could work together and strengthen institutional collaborations. Participating public libraries are discussing the possibility of developing a health information section on their websites based on the CE workshops. Albany and Troy public libraries consulted with AMC on finding health programming presenters and participated in a community event sponsored by DivCOME and the CFLJ.

The impact of the library partnerships was measured with questionnaires administered to librarians immediately after the CE workshop and three-months later. A large majority of respondents indicated that they were interested in future collaboration with Albany Medical College (82% in post-survey, 89% in three-month follow-up). Responses indicated that these collaborations may take shape as future workshops, sharing information and resources, and AMC faculty acting as advisors on future projects. When asked, "Have you or are you planning to incorporate any of the workshops' contents into your library's programming?" 56% of respondents to the three-month follow-up said "Yes" and 33% said "Maybe." Planned programming included "Medicare 101" presentations and a senior health fair including informational handouts and collaboration with community partners. One library intended to advertise that personal appointments could be made with consumer health trained librarians (see Figure 25.2).

Lessons learned

This project was, at its core, a collaboration of individuals and organizations with a shared interest in improving the health of their community members through education and empowerment. It can be replicated in settings of various sizes, locations, and target populations given those core criteria are met. Strong partnerships, institutional support, and flexibility are the keys to success (see Figure 25.3).

All five librarians who participated completed the training and received their CHIS certificates from MLA. Since then, nearly all of them have actively chosen to present programs on consumer health topics, or to participate in local consumer health events in collaboration with organizations in our area (Healthy Kids Day at the Guilderland YMCA; "Ladies Night Out" Breast Cancer Awareness Month event with the Guilderland Chamber of Commerce; programs here on yoga, making healthy snacks, etc.) All of them feel much more comfortable fielding and answering questions on health topics, and in finding the answers from excellent, reliable, current medical resources; several have actively used the iPads offered to us when doing a consultation with a patron (a very nice way to maintain privacy with an individual, since it allows us to go to a quiet room to work with that person). We're developing even more ideas, going forward, including a monthly Healthy Cookbook Club. I also can say, anecdotally, that the visibility and publicity of our health programming has attracted the attention of many clinicians and providers in the area. I regularly get calls inquiring about the possibility of presenting a program on a health topic, and the caller often cites a previous consumer health program we held.

FIGURE 25.2 GPL project impact statement.

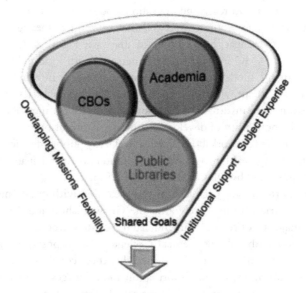

✓ Health Literacy Programs
✓ Improved Patient Physician Communication
✓ Sustainable Community Education

FIGURE 25.3 Elements of the collaboration.

Partnerships

A project of this type is only possible through the existence of strong relationships. None of the partnering organizations could have accomplished this work independently. When embarking on a similar project, the planners should leverage existing partnerships and identify possible new ones by looking for organizations that serve the populations that they are looking to target. The organizations' missions should support the overall goals. Partners should be engaged as early as possible so that they may have input throughout the planning process. During the phases of this project there was an ebb and flow of partner activity, with different partners taking a leading role at different points. The project was its most successful when the skills of all partners were leveraged. For example, the community workshops hosted at a public library but promoted by both the library and the CBO were the most well attended. Each collaboration will find its own path to success by incorporating the needs, expertise, and knowledge of those involved.

Institutional support

In addition to fostering successful partnerships with external organizations, success is dependent on the support of leadership within the sponsoring organization and each participating organization. This project involved a significant time commitment from AMC faculty. It should be noted that funds were not used to support their effort and all time on the project was in-kind. Faculty needed to work with their supervisors and coworkers to find a way to meet their responsibilities while adding the additional work required to execute this project. CBOs may not have the ability to assume the additional workload without corresponding funds for staff time. This should be considered when drafting budgets.

Flexibility

When embarking on any community outreach project, particularly one that involves a variety of partners from different organizations, flexibility is essential. At some of the community workshops attendance was significantly lower than expected, at others, three times the anticipated number of participants attended. There were changes in staff at several of the partner organizations that necessitated a shift in activities. Resources were selected based on the target audience and host location. Workshop titles should reflect session objectives to avoid misinterpretation. Misinterpretations can be sparked by current events at the local, state, national, or international level. For instance, the title "Navigating the Health Care Maze" was perceived by some attendees as a workshop about the Affordable Care Act and health insurance rather than about communicating with their healthcare providers.

Conclusion

This multi-partner collaboration demonstrates organizations with overlapping missions can work together to deliver sustainable programs that accomplish shared goals. This project is easily replicable in other communities by tailoring approaches, sites, and resources to the target population. In this case, a partnership between academia, CBOs, and public libraries allowed the project team to leverage knowledge of the target audience, skills and expertise of the partners, and understanding of the subject matter to deliver a successful program (Tables 25.1 and 25.2).

TABLE 25.1 Partnership roles and outcomes

	Academic	Community			Public Libraries
Partner	AMC–Schaffer Library of Health Sciences	AMC–Division of Community Outreach & Medical Education	Center for Law and Justice	Community Caregivers	Albany, Berne, Guilderland, Rensselaerville, Troy, Voorheesville
Setting	Urban	Urban	Urban	Suburban, rural	Urban, rural, suburban
Mission highlights	Support excellence in education, research, and patient care	Improve the health of patients; educate students and other healthcare providers on the non-biologic determinants of health	Create a fair and equitable justice system through equal access to resources; client/community empowerment; eliminating mass criminalization/incarceration; social/reparative justice	Enable individuals to maintain independence, dignity, and quality of life within their homes and communities	Provide quality library materials and services to the community for lifelong learning, cultural enrichment, and enjoyment
Populations served	Faculty, staff, students, and the general public	Students, underserved individuals, communities of color, and CBOs	Formerly incarcerated, underserved	Individuals requiring non-medical support services (mostly older adults), caregivers	General public, including underserved, minorities, elderly, disabled, caregivers

Project role	Funding oversight, project planning, expertise in health information resources, designing and leading workshops, relationship with library organizations	Project planning, relationships with CBOs, expertise in patient empowerment and communication, designing and leading workshops	Reviewing workshop content, planning community workshops (site selection, advertising)	Reviewing workshop content, planning community workshops (target audience, site selection, advertising), linking to public libraries	Recruiting 4 librarians each to attend CE workshops and receive CHIS designation, host community workshops
Outcomes	Expanded relationships with community organizations and public libraries for future outreach opportunities	Expanded relationships with community organizations and public libraries for future outreach opportunities	Increased community outreach and health education abilities Strengthened relationship with community locations used as workshop sites	Continued partnerships with libraries to expand high-quality education offerings Clarified goals for programmatic initiatives in health, aging, and wellness	Increased knowledge of resources and ability to help patrons prepare for appointments Application to programming Increased number of librarians with MLA CHIS designation

TABLE 25.2 Acronyms used

AMC	Albany Medical College
CBO	Community-Based Organization
CE	Continuing Education
CHIS	Consumer Health Information Specialization
CFLJ	Center for Law and Justice
DivCOME	Division of Community Outreach and Medical Education
MAR	Middle Atlantic Region
MLA	Medical Library Association
NNLM	National Network of Libraries of Medicine
SLHS	Schaffer Library of Health Sciences

Acknowledgment

This project has been funded in whole or in part by the National Library of Medicine (NLM), National Institutes of Health (NIH) under cooperative agreement number UG4LM012342 with the University of Pittsburgh, Health Sciences Library System.

References

American College of Obstetricians and Gynecologists. (2014). Effective patient physician communication (Committee Opinion No. 587). *Obstetrics and Gynecology, 123*, 389–93. doi:10.1097/01.AOG.0000443279.14017.12

Devine, T., Broderick, J., Harris, L. M., Wu, H., & Hilfiker, S. W. (2016). Making quality health websites a national public health priority: Towards quality standards. *Journal of Medical Internet Research, 18*, e211. doi:10.2196/jmir.5999

Fox, S., & Duggan, M. (2013). *Health online 2013.* (Pew Internet & American Life Project). Retrieved from http://www.pewinternet.org/2013/01/15/health-online-2013/

Institute of Medicine. (2004). *Health literacy: A prescription to end confusion.* Washington, DC: The National Academies Press.

Kutner, M., Greenberg, E, Jin, Y., & Paulsen, C. (2006). *The health literacy of America's adults: Results from the 2003 national assessment of adult literacy (National Center for Education Statistics–483).* Retrieved from https://nces.ed.gov/pubs2006/2006483.pdf

Pleasant, A. (2014). Advancing health literacy measurement: A pathway to better health and health system performance. *Journal of Health Communication, 19*, 1481–1496. doi:10.1080/10810730.2014.954083

United States Census Bureau. (2017). *Quick Facts.* Retrieved from https://www.census.gov/quickfacts/fact/table/saratogacountynewyork,schenectadycountynewyork,rensselaercountynewyork,albanycountynewyork/PST045217

26

TRANSFORMATIVE GLOBAL HEALTH EDUCATION AND COMMUNITY EMPOWERMENT

Moira Rogers, Robin Young, Cecilia Uribe de Chavez, and Wilfrido Torres

This chapter describes Child Family Health International (CFHI)'s long-standing Global Health education programs and community engagement practices with two key global partners, both respected leaders in their communities. Built on an asset-based community development model (Asset-Based Community Development Institute, Northwestern University, 2015), CFHI works with grassroots partners in 11 countries to develop high-quality programming for global health scholars and host communities. CFHI's global partners provide expertise in their fields through immersive learning experiences, offering visiting participants the opportunity to learn from experts and community members in the "Global South." Where many see lack of resources, CFHI recognizes resourcefulness, richness of culture, a wealth of passion, and an abundance of transformative synergies from which anyone can learn.

CFHI upholds Fair Trade Learning standards through a community-centered approach to international education and engagement. CFHI participants become "Global Ambassadors for Patient Safety" prior to undertaking global health education programs (Global Ambassadors for Patient Safety, 2015), requiring them to consider and understand the ethical role of students in the global health setting, and providing tools to reframe colonial and paternalistic approaches to global health engagement. This chapter describes lessons learned and ways of addressing challenges as opportunities for growth and deeper engagement.

The collaborations between CFHI Headquarters in San Francisco and CFHI partners in Bolivia and Ecuador have evolved over decades in response to shifting priorities and emerging needs of local communities in La Paz and Guayaquil-Puyo, of academic institutions seeking to increase global health education opportunities, and of career-focused students seeking global electives, practicums, research opportunities, and programs.

Over the past decade in the United States, a record number of students have sought global health education programs, experiences, electives, and volunteer opportunities, and more Global Health majors and minors are being offered than ever before at US academic institutions (Melby et al., 2016). This increasing demand, often driven by students' dual motivations to bolster resumes and school applications while also "doing good" or "helping the less fortunate," has brought into focus the variety in content and quality of global health education programs available to students.

There is growing concern among many in the field of Global Health Education that appropriate standards prioritizing safety, dignity, equity, and sustainability for host communities are not uniformly upheld in global health programs. Programs often prioritize participant agendas over those of host communities. Patient safety is also a major concern: The Working Group on Global Activities by Students at Pre-Health Levels has helped to document patient harm caused by students providing direct patient care and otherwise practicing medicine outside the scope of their training (Evert et al., 2015). In addition to harm to patients when students practice beyond their level or training and without knowledge of local practices, culture, language, and healthcare systems, other unintentional harms to host communities can occur when outside visitors usurp, overshadow, or do not appropriately connect their efforts to local healthcare systems and professionals. CFHI has helped to develop standards and guidelines in global health education, service-learning, and community engagement, in order to safeguard host communities and students seeking out these experiences (Evert, 2018).

To engage students in complex global health settings, it is essential that all involved – students, home institutions, and host community partners – understand students as learners, rather than volunteers filling gaps in the local healthcare system. Within the "learner" frame, students move beyond a mindset in which they may be motivated to inappropriately provide patient care (a phenomenon whose risks are now well documented) (Evert et al., 2015), or in which they see themselves as individual change-agents on short-term global health education experiences. Through pre-departure training and ongoing reflection during programs, CFHI endeavors to foster an environment in which students reflect on the privilege to immerse themselves in a global setting and learn about lasting, long-term healthcare and health initiatives under the mentorship of local experts. Recent studies have sought to understand and articulate desired competencies of students and trainees in global health settings. In 2017, individuals surveyed 170 host communities (Cherniak et al., 2017) resulting in more than 85% of respondents rating cultural awareness and respectful conduct while on a Short Term Global Health Experience (STEGH) as important. None of the respondents in this study said trainees should arrive as independent practitioners to fill healthcare gaps. Having worked with grassroots community partners since 1992, CFHI has focused on the development of program competencies that emphasize reflection, development of cultural humility and professionalism, and understanding of local culture and determinants of health. CFHI's global partners play a huge role supporting students in the development of appropriate and desirable competencies during their global health programs.

The CFHI partners featured in this chapter illustrate their rich contributions to Global Health Education for visiting participants on global health education programs, including:

- Medical and local community-based project expertise;
- Expert knowledge in their medical or public/community health field of practice;
- Deep network of community-based healthcare practitioners;
- Pedagogical expertise in cross-cultural perspectives on healthcare;
- Local networks of support (families), instructors (preceptors), and language training (language schools); and
- Rich learning field for participants to hone "soft" skills.

CFHI's US-based contributions include:

- A broad network of institutional and global health scholars enrolling in global health education programs;
- Opportunities for professional development for global partners;
- Resources (material and intellectual);
- Recruitment and enrollment management and support;
- Risk management;
- Broader advocacy and engagement to set standards around global health engagement;
- Pre-departure training and expectation setting to shift approach of participants from "volunteer" to "student/learner."

The following two examples explore health initiatives undertaken by CFHI's Medical Directors in La Paz, Bolivia, and Guayaquil and Puyo, Ecuador, to understand what the shared goals of transparency, reciprocity, equality, and sustainability look like in practice, and how visiting students and trainees fit into and appropriately support locally led initiatives.

La Paz, Bolivia: Young Women Empowerment Project (EMJ): Adolescent Mothers and Young Women in El Alto – Dr. Uribe de Chávez

Bolivia is one of the most culturally diverse countries in the world, located in the Andean Region of South America. With a population of approximately 9.1 million, 48% is of childbearing age (*Social protection in health schemes for mother, newborn and child populations: Lessons learned from the Latin American Region*, 2008). Although the country is currently undergoing a series of healthcare reforms aimed at universal health coverage through an intercultural, intersectoral, and integrated primary care system (Alvarez et al., 2016), the indigenous population continues to suffer from political and social exclusion and a 78% poverty rate, much higher than those of European descent. Maternal and infant mortality have decreased significantly, though these gains are not equally distributed, and teenage pregnancy rates remain one of the highest in Latin America (*Social protection in health schemes for mother, newborn and child populations: Lessons learned from the Latin American Region*, 2008).

Studies developed in Bolivia, focusing particularly in the city of El Alto, near La Paz, where CFHI's students spend time, illuminate the precarious situation in which young women experience their pregnancies and maternities. One study conducted at a national level (Estudio sobre el embarazo en la adolescencia en 14 municipios de Bolivia, 2016), which included El Alto, identified factors contributing to teenage pregnancies such as lack of empowerment of young women to acquire and use contraception, trusting males to handle contraception, the erroneous use of the rhythm or calendar method, and sexual violence incidents, among others.

Based on 15 years of medical practice and civil service engagement in La Paz, CFHI Medical Director adds additional contextual factors contributing to those listed above, including the adult and male-centered culture rooted in rural traditions, lack of sexual health education in schools, and limited access to contraceptive methods. Although contraception is free and widely available, taboos and other social barriers prevent young men and women from accessing it. Myths associated with the use of contraception are also an obstacle: "The Intrauterine Device causes cancer," "tubal ligation causes menstrual blood to ascend into the brain," "women who use contraceptive methods are crazy," and other myths contribute to the status quo of high rates of teenage pregnancy.

The Young Women Empowerment Project (EMJ)

Given the factors discussed earlier, the EMJ project was founded with the aim of changing perceptions and attitudes of teenage mothers who sought care at the Los Andes Hospital. This hospital is public and serves the population of the northern part of El Alto. With an emphasis on maternal-child health, 50% of women served are under the age of 24.

El Centro de Apoyo al Empoderamiento de Madres Jovenes, or EMJ (The Center for Empowerment of Young Mothers) seeks to offer women the knowledge, skills, and the opportunities to become the primary decision-makers in their own lives and thus improve the opportunities for their children. EMJ offers services including training on seeking support services for young mothers, orientation to contraceptive methods, workshops on nutrition and healthy living, vocational training, and educational support to for women looking to continue their studies. Although EMJ offers these services, resources alone cannot address the stigma that young mothers face from their partners and communities. The EMJ Center also supports women to address this stigma through workshops and case studies.

The work of the EMJ Center is challenging and requires changing deeply rooted habits and beliefs. One simple but noteworthy achievement in this project has been the wide uptake of the invisible, long-lasting, and very effective subdermal implant. During the first years of the project, all participating women chose to use the implant. The goals and projects of the EMJ Center have continued to evolve along with its participants, as the participants themselves have taken central leadership roles and articulate the services and programs they need (for example, focusing more on professional/vocational training, sexual/domestic violence, or health information). In 2017, the EMJ Center served 15 young mothers and 20 children, and transitioned to a participant-leadership model in which former participants became the primary administrators and leaders of programming.

CFHI scholars and project support

Interdisciplinary CFHI scholars at various levels have attended the CFHI Pediatric and Adolescent Medicine in La Paz program. The local hospital, under the CFHI Medical Director's leadership, a reputable teaching institution in Bolivia, has offered participants opportunities to ethically observe and discuss women and children's health with the oversight of qualified preceptors and alongside local medical students. Participants have made extensive use of library resources to prepare presentations to be discussed at grand rounds and medical debrief sessions and to nurture their reflection on their observations. Participants are referred to data and research center located in the hospital and are guided by librarians in accessing data and accessing relevant resources. Students have regularly made meaningful contributions to Quality Improvement projects at the EMJ Center, under the leadership of local administrators, through contributions to educational workshops, development of locally validated health education materials, analysis of data from the Center, and more. CFHI has invested resources to support the clinical and non-clinical sides of the Medical Director's work. After four years of support to the EMJ's project and under local leadership, the Center has found new paths for moving forward independently with sustainable funding through local partnerships. CFHI continues to send students to rotate under Medical Director Dr. Uribe's leadership, along with other key members of CFHI's local team in La Paz.

Guayaquil and Puyo, Ecuador: Promoting Community Health and Indigenous Perspectives – Dr. Torres

The Ecuadorian Constitution of 2008 declares the state as pluri-national and intercultural thus constituting a unique opportunity for the recognition and respect of all cultures as essential for the peaceful and harmonic coexistence of diverse cultures. For the past 18 years, more than 500 CFHI students have shared the daily lives of the Shuar/Kichwa community to learn about their philosophical principles and worldview, the technologies that support their practice of health, and the most relevant indigenous practices for a healthy life.

CFHI students spend time in the urban and rural areas of Guayaquil and Puyo, where they learn from experts at various levels of the healthcare system, including primary care and community health. Ecuador conceptualizes access to healthcare as the right of all citizens, a vision which has given life to programs and strategies aimed at controlling and preventing HIV, tuberculosis, Arboviri vectors (Londono-Renteria et al., 2016), safe maternity, oral health and nutrition, to name a few. These are developed with a community health approach, mobilizing the healthcare workforce to the community, balancing complex determinants of health and the interaction of humans and the environment (Londono-Renteria et al., 2016). Community Health programs are grounded in specific projects that offer tangible impacts for local communities, such as a robust, locally led diabetes project focused on teaching and research, which includes components such as taking clinical histories, trainings and workshops on nutrition, Non-Communicable Diseases (NCD's), and the use of software to track data.

Both the diabetes research project and the immersion in the Shuar/Kichwa community invite students to research and integrate scholarly findings to enrich their understanding of critical issues that shape these communities. Access to on-line resources has proven critical to teaching/learning in this program, and will continue to shape participants' perceptions of healthcare in the Global South.

Challenges and lessons learned

The partnerships described in this chapter with communities in Ecuador and Bolivia have supported the empowerment of local staff and communities, increased the prestige of preceptors and mentors within the community, and increased the perception of legitimacy for NGO's and community clinics serving marginalized populations (Richardson et al., 2016). Community partners have also reported an increase in self-awareness and perception of global citizenship, as those working with and teaching foreign visiting students understand themselves to shape participants' civic engagement, development of professional and global health competencies, and increase conscious consumption of resources. These partnerships also contribute to resource enhancement and expansion of locally led initiatives; improved local networks and leadership development for host community partners.

Several key recommendations emerge for others seeking to engage in global health education work through long-standing partnerships.

Best practices in global health engagement

Short- term Global Health Experience (STEGHs) can have serious negative impacts on host communities (Melby et al., 2016). Utilization of key frameworks such as the Fair Trade Learning Rubric, FTL, including fair allocation of resources, and developing programs rooted in existing standards is essential.

Global learning through practicums and research

In order to effectively match the needs of learners primarily from the Global North with expertise and the realities of experts and communities in the Global South, CFHI's team in San Francisco maintains an understanding of site-specific desirable competencies and areas of expertise. When students seek global health engagement for public health or global health practicums, or to support research, CFHI communicates with on-site partners to determine if students can contribute meaningfully to existing projects and objectives. Students may be able to contribute to the development of locally validated health education or outreach materials, evaluation tools, or data analysis to improve local services, for example. Students simply seeking to fulfill their own research agendas are reoriented to understand their role in the Global Health setting as one of supporting local goals and initiatives, typically through Continuous Quality Improvement (CQI). Community partners receive information and professional development from CFHI in the form of webinars, literature, and one-on-one meetings (in person and virtual) to support partner opportunities to maximally benefit from engaging students with unique or more advanced skill sets. As local realities change, CFHI works with partners to make adjustments to program design and to reimagine existing programs when local realities and priorities shift.

Navigating cross-cultural differences and facilitating complex training

Creating rich learning opportunities for diverse groups of students requires open communication channels and the ability to receive feedback and implement changes on both ends. CFHI provides intensive pre-departure training to students through various modules that focus on developing deep cultural and historical understanding of the host community; developing intercultural skills and communication tools; fostering understanding of local health realities and determinants of health; and developing an understanding of health ethics and professionalism in the global health setting.

With its global partners, CFHI engages in regular (often daily) communication and support while facilitating programs and students, as well as ongoing professional development through webinars, in-person sessions during site visits, opportunities to participate in local and global conferences, and support for individual community health projects and initiatives with accompanying capacity building as requested/needed. CFHI also recognizes the frequent lack of access to virtual libraries and journals for our global partners. We strive to regularly share open-access materials and increase access to library resources. Participants have virtual access to the library systems of their institutions and use local resources as directed by preceptors in country. In addition, CFHI keeps a rich log of articles and textbooks faculty and students refer to as they prepare for their programs.

In the management of cultural miscommunications, as well as more serious incidents and emergencies, CFHI's aim is to reach ideal outcomes by supporting our global partners who are first responders. The US-based team provides input to ensure compliance to best practices and legal regulations, while the in-country team coordinates care and response to maneuver local resources and infrastructure most effectively. It is essential to work as a respectful, collaborative team in order to ensure positive outcomes in these cases.

Participant support

Logistical and personal support of participants is essential to the success of the learning experience and requires constant monitoring and attention to feedback. Participation in community-based projects requires thorough pre-departure training to ensure students have clear and reasonable expectations about their involvement in projects and can articulate achievable outcomes.

Quality improvement

Critical to the success of CFHI's long-standing partnerships is an ongoing feedback system that allows us to understand participants' experiences and our partner's needs and challenges with the goal of establishing equitable global health partnerships. Feedback is sought both through an individual survey as well as through CFHI's participation in the Global Engagement Survey (GES; Global Engagement Survey, 2016), a multi-institutional, longitudinal study. CFHI's team in San Francisco also communicates regularly with global partners to address challenges and to collaboratively support them in their work with students.

International education and Community Engagement in global settings are complex undertakings; in no space is this truer than in global health settings. The potential risks and harms to community members are high and must remain in the forefront when offering programs for students, trainees, and other participants; in addition to the "normal" considerations of reciprocity, sustainability, transparency, and equity that should underlie any global program involving students, particularly when the directionality is North-South. CFHI's example sheds light on the centrality of framing students as learners and local leaders as experts as a baseline upon which to build long-term programs and partnerships.

References

Alvarez, F. N., Leys, M., Mérida, H. E., & Guzmán, G. E. (2016, February). Primary health care research in Bolivia: Systematic review and analysis. Retrieved from https://www.ncbi.nlm.nih.gov/pubmed/25953966

Asset-Based Community Development Institute (ABCD), Northwestern University. (2015, June 22). Retrieved from https://community-wealth.org/content/asset-based-community-development-institute-abcd-northwestern-university

Cherniak, W., Latham, E., Astle, B., Anguyo, G., Beaunoir, T., Buenaventura, J., ... Evert, J. (2017). Visiting trainees in global settings: Host and partner perspectives on desirable competencies. *Annals of Global Health, 83*(2), 359. doi:10.1016/j.aogh.2017.04.007

Estudio sobre el embarazo en la adolescencia en 14 municipios de Bolivia. (2016). Retrieved from https://bolivia.unfpa.org/sites/default/files/pub-pdf/Cartilla_Embarazo_Adolescencia_14_mun.pdf

Evert, J. (2018). Guidelines for undergraduate health-related experiences abroad. Retrieved from https://forumea.org/wp-content/uploads/2018/06/Guidelines-for-Undergraduate-Health-P3-edited.pdf

Evert, J., Todd, T., & Zitek, P. (2015). Do you GASP? How pre-health students delivering babies in Africa is quickly becoming consequentially unacceptable. *The Advisor.* Retrieved from https://www.nafsa.org/sites/default/files/ektron/files/underscore/2016colloquia/2016_health_gasp.pdf

Global Ambassadors for Patient Safety. (2015). Retrieved from https://www.healthcareers.umn.edu/courses-and-events/online-workshops/global-ambassadors-patient-safety

Global Engagement Survey (GES). (2016). Retrieved from https://compact.org/global-sl/ges/

Londono-Renteria, B., Troupin, A., & Colpitts, T. (2016, September 23). Arbovirosis and potential transmission blocking vaccines. Retrieved from https://www.ncbi.nlm.nih.gov/pmc/articles/PMC5035468/

Melby, M. K., Loh, L. C., Evert, J., Prater, C., Lin, H., & Khan, O. A. (2016). Beyond medical "missions" to impact-driven short-term experiences in global health (STEGHs). *Academic Medicine, 91*(5), 633–638. doi:10.1097/acm.0000000000001009

Richardson, E. T., Mabud, T. S., Heaney, C. A., Jones, E., Evert, J., & Kung, T. H. (2016). Host community perspectives on trainees participating in short-term experiences in global health. Retrieved from http://onlinelibrary.wiley.com/doi/10.1111/medu.13106/full

Social protection in health schemes for mother, newborn and child populations: Lessons learned from the Latin American Region. (2008). Retrieved from http://new.paho.org/hq/dmdocuments/2010/Social_Protection_Health_Schemes_MNCP.pdf

PART III

Perspectives, challenges, and future directions

27

PERSPECTIVES, CHALLENGES, AND FUTURE DIRECTIONS

Vicki Hines-Martin, Henry R. Cunningham, and Fannie M. Cox

Library Collaborations and Community Partnerships are the mechanisms by which libraries reach rural, local, regional/state, national, and global communities, as demonstrated by the exemplar's written in this book. The authors have provided a first look at the array of services, programs and initiatives that have been led by libraries to address the needs of populations and communities. Although most have been tailored to the identified needs of each setting, there are some commonalities that are evident across the different exemplars.

All exemplars clearly present the library and its interaction with library visitors as a source of initial data that served as a foundation for the resulting programming. Whether it was hunger, literacy, education, or population empowerment around an issue, the library observed that need and took action. Once that need had been identified, all authors utilized their skills as researchers to dig further for a fuller understanding of their population, the setting, resources, and strategies as an evidence-based approach to addressing a priority area.

All exemplars used a similar first step to enhance their ability to develop initiatives or programming, that of identifying what expertise they possessed. There is consistent presentation of the in-house assessment and subsequent preparation that was undertaken as each project idea was developed. Simultaneously, each project required an in-depth assessment of the strengths, talents, and resources that they did not possess which were needed to successfully undertake the efforts to meet the needs of the targeted population. Although there was variation in the amount of resources that were available internally and externally between one exemplar and another, they each made the most of those resources through seeking out available partnerships and funding where available. This identification of external resources and partners was successfully done in large part because of the broad access libraries have to databases on governmental and nongovernmental agencies, funding sources, and community organizations. Using those data, each project leader reached out to relevant entities to establish mutually beneficial collaborations. Some collaborations were interorganizational in nature and large in scope, others were interprofessional and narrowly focused in terms of targeted goals. However, all of them required partnership with defined roles as the projects progressed and evolved over time.

Throughout this book, the focus has been on addressing the needs and priorities as presented by the consumers who utilize the library and are part of the community being served. Those needs ranged from emotional wellbeing through nutrition and empowerment. Regardless of the type of programmatic approach, it was founded on the observed needs and/or priorities of the targeted population through the use of community engagement. That engagement ran the gamut from time-limited outreach to ongoing collaboration based on the goals and duration of the project.

Each of the chapters demonstrated the interactive nature of complex societal issues such as literacy and health, education, and finance, and the impact of health, education, environment, and literacy on community empowerment. These complex interactions resulted in some priority needs being discussed from different perspectives in multiple chapters; this was especially true with health and health behaviors as well as literacy. This complexity required both expected and unexpected collaborations and intervention strategies.

All contributors included efforts to evaluate the impact of their activities using qualitative and/ or quantitative methods. Some methods were more sophisticated than others. However measurement was an integral part of the process and perceptions of those involved in the process was essential including partners and recipients of their services. Data were sought regarding expected and unexpected outcomes, benefits, and challenges.

Lastly, exemplar authors all presented the work that was done as integrally a part of what a library is supposed to be and what these library staff wanted to be a part of. They demonstrated creativity, and ingenuity in both the commonplace as well as the distinctive projects that were presented. The project titles themselves were often a demonstration of this creativity.

According to the American Library Association's (ALA) Library Bill of Rights, libraries and librarians are poised to provide "free access to ideas," equal access to information for all people." Key principles of collaboration and opportunities for innovation, shared leadership, project development, and outcome measurement are all integral to this process. Capacity building for communities experiencing disparities in access and resources reflects Green's (1876) ideology of the library as a "useful institution," and using existing assets to produce applications for low-, middle-, and high-resource settings for a variety of populations is fast becoming the norm.

Various professional organizations and academic disciplines have come to recognize the importance of collaborating with librarians. Throughout this read – dependent upon the information need or societal issue – new knowledge was created; teaching, learning, and curriculum enhanced; citizens were engaged;

democratic values were strengthened; civic responsibility was exercised to impact educational attainment, health, and quality of life.

Green's four primary library functions described by Tyckoson's (2011) are still relevant in the 21st century. The field of librarianship continues to assist library users regarding how to use the library and its many resources, regardless of format. Librarians perform reference interviews to assist library users with their queries when they are not sure of what they need, to assist the user in selecting the appropriate resource(s). Last but not least, librarians act as advocates and marketer to their users, potential users, legislators/politicians, donors/philanthropist, other institutions/organizations and demonstrate how important libraries are to any community. Often, people do not know what they want or need until they need it, and then the library is the one place to start a quest for answers. As demonstrated by the various social services, professional organizations, and academic disciplines that have come to recognize the importance of collaborating with librarians, library collaborations will continue to provide non-traditional services to users of libraries.

Looking and moving forward, access to digital resources, Open Access (OA), the evolution of the Internet, technology, and social media are agents of change and represent some of the newest challenges early in the 21st century. Why challenges? Because change is constantly causing a ripple effect in expectations for discovery, bigger, better, newer technology; the acquisition of new skills, or to update old skills; adaptability, flexibility, and the willingness to learn, and all occur under the umbrella of lifelong learning. The exemplars illuminate the philosophy and perspectives that serve as a foundation for libraries and librarians as library users and libraries experience those changes.

As each of the authors note, there are challenges to partnerships and collaboration as programs and activities are developed and implemented. The challenges differ based on the nature of the projects as well as the stakeholders involved as partners. Having knowledge beforehand of the possible challenges that may be encountered when collaborating with others to address a common community issue, may help to avoid some of these pitfalls. As the exemplars demonstrate, many challenges cannot be forecast and how they are managed adds to the lessons learned column.

One of the challenges several of the projects encountered was that of logistics. Some of the logistical issues involved scheduling, staffing, and location among others. Scheduling appears to be the biggest hurdle that partners needed to overcome. With different stakeholders at the table with their varied schedules, it became difficult in some cases to schedule activities at times convenient for everyone. In some cases, holidays and other work schedules impacted deadlines of program implementation and completion as noted with one project. At other times, partners indicated they had to juggle speakers' availability, facilities, and the most convenient time to reach participants as they worked on scheduling events. Challenges can be as simple as getting children to the site, so while scheduling might be convenient for both the children and facilitators to hold an event during the day, in some cases events had to be held in the evenings when parents drive children to and from the event. The same issues apply to programs with seniors, finding the time that works for them needed to be explored.

Location is another logistical issue that was experienced by partners. Not only must the site location be convenient for participants to access but it must also be convenient to others who may be affected as well. In one such case, the library setting was an ideal venue to host a yoga class but the noise from the class affected other patrons at the library. This particular challenge was not anticipated and created logistical issues for organizers. Finding the appropriate location for certain services can sometimes also be a challenge. While the idea of a community garden sounded like a good one to engage the community, the site of the garden was not within walking distance and with no available transportation, the idea had to be abandoned. The weather can also create its own logistical nightmare if outdoor activities are scheduled on cold or rainy days.

For one project, the concern revolved around legal issues. There was the concern of liability in the case of injury to participants in the program. There is also the issue of taking children off library property for an activity. The question becomes what happens if one of the children is hurt and who is responsible? Not only can the legal ramification be worrisome but it may cause some individuals to be hesitant in engaging in certain activities.

When coordinating programs, it is necessary to have the staffing to carry out the activities. While many libraries and community organizations may depend on volunteers to assist with its work, permanent staff serves as the core of the organization. This was an issue with several libraries and community partners, which experienced staff turnover in the midst of a program. This loss of expertise and experience may slow implementation of a project or halt the work altogether. When remaining staff members must fill in for those who departed, this has the potential to result in some work not getting full attention as staff members find themselves stretched thin. In other cases, the staff may just not have enough time to devote to certain initiatives. In one instance, staff members indicated that they felt overwork and experienced burn out. This becomes a staff scheduling challenge, an issue experienced by several libraries, which are featured in this book.

Another major challenge experienced by several libraries in collaborating with community partners were the cultural issues that surfaced, some of which were unexpected. Issues such as language barriers, whereby monolingual staff are dealing with individuals from the community who are not well versed in English. While bilingual staff members and volunteers serving as interpreters and translators can be of assistance, other issues such as explaining complex terminology and concepts in another language may pose a problem for library staff.

Similarly, the issue of cross-cultural sensitivity can be a challenge, particularly when working in a community whose culture is distinctly different from those of the service providers. This challenge may be magnified ten-fold when working in another country, as was the case of those from Child Family Health International who worked in Bolivia and Ecuador. Such situations require navigating cross-cultural differences when working with members of the host country. It is important to respect the beliefs, customs, and traditions of the community and be very sensitive to these situations. Beliefs and customs are deep-rooted and one must be mindful of that to best collaborate with members of the community. Such challenges need to be addressed upfront with proper and extensive cross-cultural training prior to the beginning of any work in such communities.

In other cases, cultural sensitivity is necessary when dealing with controversial topics such as sex education. While sex education is offered in some schools, some parents even discuss sex with their children to better educate them on the topic. For others, it is a taboo topic. This was a challenge for one library and its staff, who were engaged in a sex education program for youth. What is noteworthy about how this project was implemented is that organizers involved the youth in marketing the sex education classes. Their rational for doing this is that the youngsters understand the language of their peers and that of their parents and therefore more likely to use more appropriate terms in marketing the classes to them. The project leaders also developed a script to respond to any concerns that might be expressed by parents.

For many of the libraries, the concept of how to partner with community stakeholders or how partners collaborate with the library was something with which many of them had to grapple. This particular challenge arose when it was discovered that not all partners understood the partnership process. As Morey, Comtois, and Panagakis noted in this volume, partnership required interdependence. It is a collaborative effort and therefore, partners cannot be independent of each other but must work together toward a common goal. An integral part of collaboration is communication which some also viewed as a challenge. How do we keep everyone abreast of what is happening, particularly as it related to changes and new information? Good communication was noted as important to the partnership as it helps to build trust among collaborators and the population being served.

One challenge noted as part of the partnering process was the ability to find other libraries with similar missions with which to partner, that is, a library with an outreach mission. Having a common interest such as community outreach makes the collaboration much easier. Similarly, the project that is undertaken must be mutually beneficial to all stakeholders. In one instance as noted by Russo, students from the university involved in a service-learning or community-based learning course with the local public library were prevented from having meaningful interaction with library visitors which is a key element in community engagement as mutual benefit is an important aspect of partnership, collaboration, and service-learning.

Other challenges encountered in the partnership between libraries and their stakeholders included difficulty with assessing impact of the work. In-depth impact assessment can be a challenge if you do not have the expertise on your staff or the time for it to be conducted. A few libraries had difficulty assessing collaborative efforts because of the issues raised. The issue of program sustainability over the long term is also something some libraries and their partners experienced. This was more of a concern for those programs that were grant funded. The issue of sustainability was also a concern for those programs that were led by individuals within the organization who were not in a leadership role within the organization. There is concern of what happens should that point person leave since leadership is not invested or involved in the project.

The challenges encountered provided a great learning opportunity for many stakeholders. Authors of the chapters discussed the many lessons learned from the challenges, which helped to enhance program offerings. Despite the challenges, there was much success to celebrate. There were positive outcomes from all the projects that strengthened communities in many ways. Programs were implemented, thus enhancing the quality of life of community residents through education, providing tools to help communities improve health behaviors and transforming others through social and financial skill development. These partnerships and collaborations helped to build bridges among community stakeholders, both libraries and community organizations, and helped to improve the perception of libraries in addressing critical community needs.

As authors described their processes, outcomes, challenges, and lessons learned, they also presented some overarching recommendations for the future.

- Promote the idea that problem solving and innovation are key aspects of library functioning
- Utilize the resources not only of the library but also the community to build capacity
- Recognize the importance of communication; not only with library users but with a variety of others to build relationships, partnerships, and function as advocates for those being served
- Grow the research about library-led projects to build the evidence base about their impact
- Share the stories of library projects and shine a light on successful contributions to demonstrate the many possibilities and enlighten those considering library science as a vocation or those individuals wishing to expand their efforts, in collaboration with other professions and stakeholders.

References

Green, S. S. (1876). Personal relations between librarians and readers. *Library Journal, 1*, 74–81.

Tyckoson, D. A. (2011). Issues and trends in the management of reference services: A historical perspective. *Journal of Library Administration, 51*(3), 259–278, doi:10.1080/01 930826.2011.556936

INDEX

Note: **bold** page numbers refer to tables and *italic* page numbers refer to figures.

Printed in the United States
by Baker & Taylor Publisher Services